# Psychiatric Medications Made Simple

A Practical Psychopharmacology Guide for Mental Health Clinicians

Charles Tadelesh Prada and Judith Victoria Perkins

ISBN: 978-1-7641942-0-4

Isohan Publishing

# Table of Contents

**Chapter 1: How Psych Meds Work** ................................................ 1

The Brain as a Communication Network .................................. 1

Key Neurotransmitter Systems ................................................ 2

How Medications Change Brain Chemistry .......................... 4

Clinical Vignette: Sarah's First Antidepressant ................. 5

Moving Forward with Understanding ................................... 6

**Chapter 2: The Clinician's Role in Medication Management** .......... 8

The Split Treatment Model .................................................... 8

Recognizing Medication Effects ......................................... 10

Patient Education Fundamentals ........................................ 12

Documentation and Communication .................................. 14

Case Study: Managing a Patient Across Multiple Providers ..... 15

**Bridging Knowledge and Practice** ................................ 16

**Chapter 3: Safety First: Critical Concepts** ................................ 18

Drug Interactions Simplified ................................................ 18

Special Populations Overview ............................................. 20

Emergency Situations ........................................................... 23

Clinical Vignette: Recognizing Serotonin Syndrome in the Therapy Office ..................................................................... 25

Quick Reference Box: Emergency Contact Protocols ............. 26

Staying Vigilant .................................................................... 27

**Chapter 4: Antidepressants - Lifting the Fog** ............................ 29

SSRIs: The First-Line Warriors ............................................ 29

Case Vignette: John's Journey from Lexapro to Zoloft ........... 31

SNRIs: The Dual-Action Approach ...................................... 32

Atypical Antidepressants: The Specialists ......................... 34

Case Study: Choosing the Right Antidepressant for Maria........35

Older Antidepressants: Still Relevant .......................................36

Moving Forward with Antidepressant Knowledge ...................38

**Chapter 5: Mood Stabilizers - Finding Balance ........................ 40**

Lithium: The Gold Standard.......................................................40

Case Vignette: Sarah's Lithium Success Story.........................42

Anticonvulsants as Mood Stabilizers ........................................43

Case Study: Transitioning from Lithium to Lamotrigine...........46

Combination Strategies ...............................................................47

Achieving Stability Through Understanding..............................48

**Chapter 6: Antipsychotics - Beyond Psychosis........................ 50**

Understanding Antipsychotics.....................................................50

Clinical Uses Beyond Schizophrenia ........................................51

Case Vignette: Using Abilify for Treatment-Resistant
Depression ...................................................................................52

Managing Metabolic Effects ......................................................53

Movement Disorders: Recognition and Response ....................56

Case Study: Recognizing and Addressing Akathisia ................58

Practical Wisdom for Antipsychotic Use ..................................59

**Chapter 7: Anxiety Medications - Calming the Storm................... 61**

Benzodiazepines: Benefits and Risks.........................................61

Case Vignette: Helping James Taper Off Xanax .....................64

Alternative Anxiolytics ...............................................................65

Case Study: Choosing Non-Addictive Anxiety Treatment ........67

Building Comprehensive Treatment............................................68

**Chapter 8: Specialty Medications ............................................. 70**

ADHD Medications.....................................................................70

Case Example 1: The Struggling Student ................................ 72

Sleep Medications ................................................................ 74

Case Vignette: Addressing Chronic Insomnia Safely ............... 76

Cognitive Enhancers ............................................................ 77

Case Example 2: Managing Expectations ................................ 79

Practical Perspectives on Specialty Medications ..................... 80

**Chapter 9: Drug Interactions and Safety ............................82**

CYP450 System Simplified .................................................... 82

Case Example 1: The Dangerous Combination ......................... 84

Serotonin Syndrome Deep Dive.............................................. 85

Case Example 2: The Supplement Surprise .............................. 87

QT Prolongation: The Heart Rhythm Risk ............................... 88

Clinical Scenarios: Interaction Management in Practice ........... 89

Case Example 3: The Hidden Interaction ................................ 91

Building Systematic Safcty .................................................. 92

**Chapter 10: Special Populations in Detail .........................94**

Pregnancy and Breastfeeding................................................. 94

Case Study: Managing Bipolar Disorder in Pregnancy ............. 96

Children and Adolescents .................................................... 97

Case Example 1: The Activated Adolescent .............................. 99

Geriatric Considerations....................................................... 100

Case Example 2: The Complex Elderly Patient ...................... 102

Case Example 3: The Pregnant Professional ......................... 103

Adapting Treatment for Success ........................................... 104

**Chapter 11: Practical Clinical Scenarios .........................106**

Treatment-Resistant Depression: Step-by-Step Approaches ... 106

Case Example 1: Breaking Through Resistance ...................... 108

Managing Non-adherence: Real-World Strategies.................. 108

Case Example 2: The Ambivalent Patient............................... 110

Emergency Situations: Office-Based Responses..................... 111

Complex Cases: Multiple Diagnoses, Multiple Medications .. 112

Case Example 3: The Complex Case Conference................... 113

Cultural Considerations: Adapting Approaches...................... 114

Integrating All Elements.......................................................... 116

**Chapter 12: Essential References ...............................................118**

Medication Comparison Tables................................................ 118

Case Example 1: The Confusing Consultation........................ 121

Dosing Quick Guides .............................................................. 122

Monitoring Checklists .............................................................. 124

Case Example 2: The Missed Monitoring............................... 126

Patient Education Templates .................................................... 127

Case Example 3: The Educational Success ............................. 129

Emergency Contact Protocols .................................................. 130

Building Your Personal Reference System ............................. 131

**Reference ...........................................................................................133**

# Chapter 1: How Psych Meds Work

The human brain contains approximately 86 billion neurons, each one forming thousands of connections with other neurons. This vast network processes every thought, emotion, and behavior through chemical messages that zip between cells at lightning speed. When these chemical conversations go awry, mental health symptoms emerge. Understanding how psychiatric medications work starts with grasping this fundamental communication system—not through complex neuroscience jargon, but through simple, practical analogies that make sense in everyday clinical practice.

## The Brain as a Communication Network

Think of your brain as a massive telephone network where billions of cells need to talk to each other constantly. Each neuron acts like a telephone line, carrying messages from one point to another. But unlike phone calls that use electrical signals through wires, brain cells communicate through chemicals called neurotransmitters—the actual "messages" being sent.

Between each neuron lies a tiny gap called a synapse, which functions as a conversation space where these chemical messages get passed along. Imagine two people having a conversation across a small table at a coffee shop. The person speaking (the presynaptic neuron) releases words (neurotransmitters) that travel across the table (synapse) to reach the listener's ears (receptors on the postsynaptic neuron). This conversation happens billions of times per second throughout your brain.

Psychiatric medications work by changing these conversations in specific ways. Some medications make the speaker talk louder or more frequently. Others might plug the listener's ears partially, turning down the volume. Still others might keep the words hanging in the air longer, extending the conversation. By understanding these basic mechanisms, clinicians can better explain to patients how their medications work and why certain side effects occur.

1

## Case Example 1: The Anxious Executive

Jennifer, a 42-year-old marketing executive, sits in your office describing her constant worry and racing thoughts. "My brain won't shut off," she says. You explain: "Your brain cells are having conversations using a chemical called GABA—think of it as your brain's natural brake pedal. With anxiety, it's like driving a car where the brakes aren't working well. The anti-anxiety medication your doctor prescribed helps your brain cells hear the GABA messages better, essentially fixing those brakes so your thoughts can slow down when needed."

This simple explanation helps Jennifer understand why her medication works and why she needs to take it regularly—the brakes need consistent maintenance to function properly.

## Key Neurotransmitter Systems

The brain uses dozens of different neurotransmitters, but five major systems account for most psychiatric symptoms and medication effects. Each system has distinct functions, and understanding them helps predict both therapeutic effects and side effects.

**Serotonin serves as the mood stabilizer system.** Picture serotonin as a thermostat that keeps your emotional temperature steady. When serotonin levels drop or its signaling falters, mood swings occur—depression creeps in like a cold draft, anxiety builds like overheating, and sleep patterns become erratic. Most antidepressants work primarily on this system, which explains why they help with mood, anxiety, and sleep issues simultaneously (1).

**Dopamine functions as the reward and reality system.** This neurotransmitter creates feelings of pleasure and motivation while also helping maintain our grip on reality. Too little dopamine in certain brain areas leads to the flat emotions and lack of motivation seen in depression. Too much in other areas can trigger the hallucinations and delusions of psychosis. This dual role explains why some medications that block dopamine help psychosis but can cause depression-like symptoms as side effects (2).

**Norepinephrine acts as the alertness and energy system.** Like an alarm clock for your brain, norepinephrine keeps you awake, alert, and ready for action. Low levels contribute to the fatigue and poor concentration common in depression. High levels fuel the physical symptoms of anxiety—racing heart, sweating, and that jittery feeling. Medications that boost norepinephrine can improve energy but might worsen anxiety in some patients (3).

**GABA operates as the brake pedal system.** This inhibitory neurotransmitter slows down brain activity wherever it's released. Without enough GABA activity, the brain races like a car with no brakes—leading to anxiety, seizures, and insomnia. Medications that enhance GABA, like benzodiazepines, provide rapid relief for anxiety but can make people feel mentally slowed or sedated (4).

**Glutamate works as the accelerator pedal system.** As the brain's main excitatory neurotransmitter, glutamate speeds up brain activity and plays crucial roles in learning and memory. Problems with glutamate signaling contribute to various psychiatric conditions, from depression to schizophrenia. Some newer medications target this system, offering hope for patients who don't respond to traditional treatments (5).

### Case Example 2: The Tired Teacher

Mark, a 35-year-old high school teacher, struggles with severe depression. Despite trying two different SSRIs (which mainly target serotonin), he remains exhausted and unmotivated. His psychiatrist switches him to bupropion, explaining it works on dopamine and norepinephrine instead. You reinforce this in therapy: "The previous medications were fixing your mood thermostat, but your brain's alarm clock and reward systems still needed help. This new medication targets those specific systems, which is why you're finally getting your energy back."

Understanding these distinctions helps Mark make sense of his treatment journey and reduces his frustration about the initial medication failures.

## How Medications Change Brain Chemistry

Psychiatric medications alter brain chemistry through three main mechanisms, each easily understood through everyday analogies that patients can grasp and remember.

**Reuptake inhibitors work like drain plugs.** After neurotransmitters deliver their message across the synapse, the sending cell usually vacuums them back up through reuptake pumps—like water going down a drain. Reuptake inhibitors plug these drains, keeping more neurotransmitter in the synapse to continue the conversation. This mechanism explains how SSRIs (selective serotonin reuptake inhibitors) increase serotonin activity without actually producing more serotonin (6).

**Receptor blockers function as door locks.** These medications attach to receptors on the receiving cell, preventing neurotransmitters from binding—like changing the locks on a door so the original key no longer works. Antipsychotic medications use this mechanism to block dopamine receptors, reducing psychotic symptoms. However, because dopamine has many jobs throughout the brain, blocking its receptors can cause various side effects (7).

**Enzyme inhibitors shut down recycling plants.** Enzymes in the brain break down used neurotransmitters for recycling. Some medications inhibit these enzymes, allowing neurotransmitters to accumulate. MAO inhibitors work this way, preventing the breakdown of serotonin, norepinephrine, and dopamine. This powerful effect explains both their effectiveness and their potential for dangerous interactions (8).

**Case Example 3: The Reluctant Patient**

4

David, a 28-year-old software developer, expresses skepticism about starting an antidepressant. "I don't want some drug changing who I am," he says. You explain: "Think of depression like a clogged sink that's not draining properly. The medication doesn't add anything foreign—it just unplugs the drain so your brain's natural chemicals can flow the way they're supposed to. You're still you, just with better plumbing."

This concrete analogy helps David understand that SSRIs work with his brain's existing chemistry rather than replacing it with something artificial.

## Clinical Vignette: Sarah's First Antidepressant

Sarah, a 34-year-old nurse, arrives at her therapy appointment two weeks after starting sertraline for depression and anxiety. She looks worried and pulls out her phone, showing you a list of side effects she's been tracking.

"I've had some nausea, my sleep is weird, and I actually feel more anxious," she says. "Is this normal? Should I stop taking it?"

You lean forward with reassurance. "What you're experiencing makes perfect sense when you understand what's happening in your brain right now. Let me explain it simply."

Drawing a basic diagram, you continue: "Your brain cells communicate using serotonin—think of it as text messages between cells. Depression happens when these messages aren't getting through clearly. The sertraline works by keeping these messages available longer, like preventing texts from being deleted too quickly."

"But here's what's happening in your first few weeks: Your brain cells aren't used to having so many messages available. Some cells are getting overwhelmed—that's causing your nausea and anxiety. Others are adjusting their sensitivity—affecting your sleep. Your brain is essentially recalibrating its communication system."

Sarah nods, beginning to understand. "So these side effects mean it's working?"

"Exactly. Most patients experience what you're describing in the first two to three weeks. The side effects typically fade as your brain adjusts, while the benefits for mood and anxiety build gradually over four to six weeks. Think of it like starting a new exercise routine— you feel sore at first, but that discomfort leads to getting stronger."

You provide her with specific strategies: taking the medication with food for nausea, temporarily moving her dose to bedtime if it makes her drowsy, and using the relaxation techniques you've practiced for managing the temporary anxiety increase.

"What warning signs should I watch for?" Sarah asks, showing her clinical knowledge.

"You're right to ask. While these side effects are expected, call your prescriber immediately if you experience severe symptoms like extreme agitation, confusion, fever, or suicidal thoughts. Those could indicate rare but serious reactions."

Three weeks later, Sarah reports significant improvement. The nausea resolved completely, her anxiety decreased below her baseline, and her mood lifted noticeably. "Understanding what was happening in my brain made all the difference," she reflects. "I might have stopped taking it without your explanation."

## Moving Forward with Understanding

Psychiatric medications work by fine-tuning the chemical conversations happening in your brain every moment. Rather than mysteriously altering personality or artificially creating emotions, these medications simply adjust how brain cells communicate with each other. This fundamental understanding empowers both clinicians and patients to approach medication treatment as a collaborative process based on brain science rather than trial-and-error guesswork.

The key lies in translating complex neuroscience into practical understanding. When patients grasp how their medications work, they're more likely to take them correctly, tolerate initial side effects, and communicate effectively with their treatment team. As you continue through this guide, you'll build on these foundational concepts to understand specific medication classes and their clinical applications

**Key Takeaways**

- The brain functions as a vast communication network where neurons exchange chemical messages across synapses
- Five major neurotransmitter systems (serotonin, dopamine, norepinephrine, GABA, and glutamate) govern most psychiatric symptoms
- Medications work through three main mechanisms: blocking reuptake (drain plugs), blocking receptors (door locks), or inhibiting enzymes (shutting down recycling plants)
- Understanding these basic mechanisms helps predict both therapeutic effects and side effects
- Using simple analogies improves patient understanding and medication adherence
- Early side effects often indicate the medication is beginning to work and typically improve with time

# Chapter 2: The Clinician's Role in Medication Management

Mental health treatment increasingly involves team-based care, with different professionals contributing their unique expertise. As a non-prescribing clinician, you occupy a crucial position in this ecosystem—often spending more time with patients than prescribers do, observing medication effects in real-world contexts, and building the trust necessary for honest communication about symptoms and side effects. Your role extends far beyond simply referring patients for medication evaluation; you serve as an educator, monitor, advocate, and bridge between patients and prescribers.

## The Split Treatment Model

Modern mental health care frequently involves "split treatment," where one professional provides psychotherapy while another manages medications. This model creates both opportunities and challenges that require careful navigation to ensure optimal patient outcomes.

**When you're not the prescriber,** your observations become invaluable data points. You see patients weekly or biweekly, noticing subtle changes in mood, behavior, and functioning that might escape detection in brief medication appointments every few months. You hear about side effects patients hesitate to mention to prescribers, witness medication effects on family dynamics, and observe real-world functioning between appointments.

Consider the difference in contact: A psychiatrist might see a patient for 15-20 minutes every three months for medication management. You might spend 50 minutes weekly with that same patient. Over three months, that's approximately 10 hours of clinical contact versus 20 minutes—a 30-fold difference in observation time. This disparity makes your input essential for optimal medication management (9).

**Collaborative care essentials** require establishing clear communication channels while respecting professional boundaries. Successful collaboration starts with obtaining proper releases of information and establishing preferred communication methods with prescribers. Some prefer brief emails highlighting specific concerns. Others want structured updates using standardized forms. Many appreciate phone calls for urgent issues but written communication for routine updates.

Your communications should focus on observable behaviors and functional changes rather than diagnostic opinions or medication recommendations. For instance, instead of suggesting "the patient needs a higher dose," you might report: "The patient continues to miss 2-3 days of work weekly due to depressive symptoms despite 6 weeks on current medication dose. Sleep remains fragmented with 3-4 awakenings nightly, and concentration problems interfere with job tasks."

## Case Example 1: The Overlooked Side Effect

Tom, a 45-year-old accountant, sees his psychiatrist quarterly for bipolar disorder management. During therapy, you notice he's developed a subtle hand tremor and seems to drink water constantly. When asked, he admits, "Yeah, the shaking is annoying, especially when I'm trying to use the computer. And I'm in the bathroom every hour—it's embarrassing during client meetings."

He hadn't mentioned these lithium side effects to his psychiatrist, assuming they were "just part of taking medication." Your email to the prescriber detailed the functional impact: "Patient reports fine motor tremor interfering with typing (job essential) and urinary frequency requiring hourly bathroom breaks during 2-hour client meetings. Both symptoms began approximately 4 weeks after lithium increase."

The psychiatrist responded by ordering lithium levels and ultimately adjusted the dosing schedule, significantly improving both side effects while maintaining mood stability.

**Communication with prescribers** works best when you establish mutual respect and clear roles. Effective messages are concise, specific, and focused on functional observations. They include relevant timelines, specific examples, and clear descriptions of impact on daily functioning. Avoid psychiatric jargon when simple descriptions work better, and always distinguish between patient reports and your observations (10).

A well-crafted communication might read: "During the past 3 sessions, patient has shown marked psychomotor retardation—taking 5-10 seconds to respond to questions, moving slowly when entering/leaving office. Patient reports requiring 2+ hours each morning to complete basic self-care. Started approximately 2 weeks after beginning risperidone. No previous psychomotor symptoms observed in 6 months of treatment."

## Recognizing Medication Effects

Your regular contact with patients positions you to notice medication effects—both therapeutic and adverse—that might otherwise go unrecognized. Understanding typical response patterns helps you provide accurate feedback to prescribers and realistic expectations to patients.

**Therapeutic response timelines** vary significantly between medication classes and individual patients. Antidepressants typically require 4-6 weeks for full effect, though some patients notice subtle improvements within 2 weeks. Sleep and appetite often improve before mood lifts. Anxiety might temporarily worsen before improving. Antipsychotics can reduce agitation within hours but may take weeks to fully address psychotic symptoms. Mood stabilizers show different timelines for acute symptoms versus prevention of future episodes (11).

Understanding these patterns helps you support patients through the challenging early weeks of treatment. When someone says, "This medication isn't working" after 10 days on an SSRI, you can provide informed reassurance while documenting their specific concerns for the prescriber.

**Side effect identification** requires active inquiry since patients often don't spontaneously report problems they assume are unchangeable. Sexual dysfunction affects up to 70% of patients on SSRIs but goes unreported in most cases due to embarrassment. Weight gain creeps up gradually, making it easy to miss without regular monitoring. Cognitive dulling from mood stabilizers might manifest as work performance problems before patients recognize the connection (12).

Your therapeutic relationship creates safe space for these difficult conversations. Simple questions like "Have you noticed any changes in your physical health since starting this medication?" or "How's your energy and focus at work these days?" can uncover significant side effects affecting quality of life.

**Case Example 2: The Gradual Decline**

Maria, a 38-year-old teacher, had taken paroxetine successfully for anxiety for two years. Over several months, you noticed subtle changes: arriving to sessions looking disheveled, forgetting appointment times, seeming less engaged in conversations. When explored, she revealed: "I just feel... foggy. Like I'm thinking through cotton. My principal commented on mistakes in my lesson plans."

Further discussion revealed she'd gained 30 pounds, felt constantly fatigued, and had lost interest in sex—all gradual changes she'd attributed to "getting older" rather than medication effects. Your detailed communication to her psychiatrist led to a medication switch to bupropion, ultimately restoring her cognitive clarity and energy while maintaining anxiety control.

**Red flags requiring immediate attention** include symptoms suggesting potentially dangerous adverse reactions. Serotonin syndrome can develop when medications affecting serotonin combine or doses increase too rapidly. Watch for agitation, confusion, rapid heart rate, dilated pupils, muscle rigidity, or high fever. Neuroleptic malignant syndrome from antipsychotics presents with severe muscle rigidity, fever, and altered consciousness. Severe allergic reactions might begin with rashes that spread or involve mucous membranes (13).

Your role isn't to diagnose these conditions but to recognize warning signs and facilitate immediate medical attention. Having prescriber emergency contacts readily available and knowing when to recommend emergency department evaluation can save lives.

## Patient Education Fundamentals

Effective patient education about medications requires translating complex medical information into understandable, practical guidance. Your ongoing relationship allows for education spread across multiple sessions, reinforcing key concepts and addressing concerns as they arise.

**Using plain language effectively** means avoiding medical jargon while maintaining accuracy. Instead of "This medication inhibits serotonin reuptake," try "This medication helps your brain's mood chemicals work more effectively by keeping them active longer." Rather than discussing "anticholinergic effects," explain "This medication might cause dry mouth, constipation, and blurry vision because it affects the nerve signals controlling these functions" (14).

Create mental pictures that stick. Describe extended-release medications as "like a timed-release vitamin that slowly dissolves throughout the day" rather than using technical terms. Explain half-lives using analogies: "If you skip a dose of this medication, it's like your brain's thermostat slowly drifting back to its old setting over several days."

**Common patient concerns and responses** follow predictable patterns. Fear of addiction tops the list, especially with anxiety medications. Distinguish between physical dependence (the body adapting to a medication) and addiction (compulsive use despite harm). Explain: "Your body might adjust to this medication like it adjusts to caffeine—you'd feel different if you stopped suddenly. But

12

that's not addiction, which involves craving and harmful behavior" (15).

Worries about personality changes require careful attention. Patients often ask, "Will I still be myself?" Address this directly: "Psychiatric medications don't create new personalities or emotions. They help your brain chemistry work more like it does when you're feeling your best. You're still you—just without symptoms holding you back."

## Case Example 3: The Ambivalent Artist

James, a 26-year-old graphic designer, worried that antidepressants would destroy his creativity. "All my best work comes from intense emotions," he insisted. "What if medication makes me a boring robot?"

You addressed his concern thoughtfully: "Many creative people share your worry. Research actually shows that treating depression often enhances creativity by improving focus and energy. The medication doesn't eliminate emotions—it prevents them from becoming so overwhelming that they paralyze you. Think of it like cleaning smudges off your glasses. You see the same world, just more clearly."

You also connected him with other artists who'd successfully used psychiatric medications, normalizing his concerns while providing real-world reassurance. Three months later, James reported completing more projects than in the previous year, with improved quality and client satisfaction.

**Adherence strategies that work** go beyond simple reminders to take medication. Help patients identify personal motivations for treatment success. Link medication adherence to their specific goals: returning to work, being present for children, enjoying hobbies again. Create behavioral chains connecting medication-taking to established routines—morning coffee, brushing teeth, or feeding pets (16).

Address practical barriers proactively. If cost concerns arise, research patient assistance programs or discuss generic alternatives with prescribers. For complex regimens, help create visual medication schedules or recommend pill organizers. When side effects interfere with adherence, work with patients to identify which effects they can tolerate versus those requiring medication adjustments.

## Documentation and Communication

Proper documentation protects patients, supports clinical decision-making, and facilitates team coordination. Your notes create a detailed record of medication responses that prescribers rely upon for treatment planning.

**What to document** includes both objective observations and subjective patient reports. Note medication names, doses, and timing of changes. Record specific symptoms and their severity using consistent language. Document functional impacts: work attendance, social engagement, self-care abilities. Track side effects with onset timing and severity. Include patient attitudes toward medications and adherence patterns (17).

Effective documentation uses specific behavioral descriptions. Instead of "patient seems manic," write: "Patient spoke rapidly without pause for first 20 minutes of session, reported sleeping 2-3 hours nightly for past week, described starting three new business ventures since last session. Pressured speech noted with flight of ideas between topics."

**HIPAA-compliant communication** requires careful attention to privacy regulations while maintaining necessary information flow. Use secure email systems or encrypted platforms for written communications. Avoid patient identifiers in subject lines. When leaving voicemails, state only your name and request a return call without mentioning patient information. Fax communications only to verified numbers with cover sheets marked confidential (18).

**Emergency protocols** should be established proactively with clear escalation procedures. Know which situations warrant immediate prescriber contact versus next-business-day communication. Maintain current emergency contact information for prescribers, including coverage arrangements. Understand your prescribers' preferences for

14

after-hours contact—some provide cell phones for emergencies while others prefer emergency department referral with follow-up notification.

Create written protocols for common scenarios: suspected serotonin syndrome, acute dystonic reactions, severe mood episodes, or suicidal ideation with medication changes. Having clear procedures reduces anxiety and improves response time during crises.

## Case Study: Managing a Patient Across Multiple Providers

Lisa, a 52-year-old divorced mother of two, exemplifies the complexities of modern mental health care. She sees you weekly for therapy addressing PTSD from childhood trauma, meets with a psychiatrist monthly for medication management of bipolar disorder, and recently started seeing a primary care physician who prescribed gabapentin for fibromyalgia.

During a routine therapy session, Lisa mentions feeling "strange" lately. Through careful questioning, you discover she's experiencing mild euphoria, decreased sleep, and increased goal-directed activity—possible early hypomanic symptoms. She also reports dizziness and mild confusion, particularly in the mornings.

Your investigation reveals a complex situation: Lisa's psychiatrist recently increased her lamotrigine dose for better depression control. Her primary care physician, unaware of the dose change, prescribed gabapentin which can interact with lamotrigine. Additionally, Lisa started taking over-the-counter St. John's Wort for "natural mood support," not realizing it could trigger mania and interact with her psychiatric medications.

Your response demonstrates coordinated care at its best:

1. **Immediate safety assessment**: Confirming Lisa wasn't experiencing severe symptoms requiring emergency intervention

15

2. **Patient education**: Explaining medication interactions in understandable terms and the importance of informing all providers about all medications, including supplements
3. **Coordinated communication**: With Lisa's consent, you contact both prescribers:
   - Email to psychiatrist detailing observed hypomanic symptoms with specific behavioral examples and timeline
   - Call to primary care physician explaining psychiatric medication regimen and potential interaction concerns
4. **Documentation**: Detailed session notes including all medications, observed symptoms, patient education provided, and communications with providers
5. **Follow-up planning**: Scheduling increased session frequency for monitoring and creating a medication reconciliation system for Lisa to share with all providers

The psychiatrist responded by temporarily reducing lamotrigine, discontinuing St. John's Wort, and coordinating with the primary care physician about gabapentin timing to minimize interactions. Your observations and coordination prevented potential mood destabilization while maintaining treatment for Lisa's chronic pain.

This case illustrates how non-prescribing clinicians serve as vital connectors in fragmented healthcare systems, catching potentially dangerous situations through careful observation and facilitating communication between providers who might otherwise work in isolation.

## Bridging Knowledge and Practice

Your unique position in the treatment team—combining frequent patient contact with clinical expertise—makes you an invaluable asset in medication management. By recognizing medication effects, providing informed patient education, maintaining clear documentation, and facilitating team communication, you significantly improve treatment outcomes. The key lies not in becoming a medication expert but in leveraging your therapeutic relationship to support optimal medication use while maintaining appropriate professional boundaries.

**Key Takeaways**

- Non-prescribing clinicians see patients more frequently than prescribers, providing crucial observations about medication effects and side effects
- Effective collaboration requires clear communication focusing on specific behaviors and functional impacts rather than diagnostic opinions
- Understanding medication response timelines helps set realistic expectations and identify when interventions are needed
- Patient education using plain language and relatable analogies improves medication adherence and reduces anxiety
- Systematic documentation creates valuable records for treatment planning and team coordination
- Proactive emergency protocols and clear escalation procedures improve crisis response
- Coordinating care across multiple providers prevents dangerous interactions and improves outcomes

# Chapter 3: Safety First: Critical Concepts

Safety in psychopharmacology extends beyond avoiding adverse reactions—it encompasses understanding drug interactions, recognizing vulnerable populations, and responding effectively to emergencies. While prescribers bear primary responsibility for medication safety, non-prescribing clinicians serve as essential safety monitors, often catching problems before they escalate into crises. Your frequent patient contact and therapeutic relationship create unique opportunities to identify safety concerns that might otherwise go unnoticed until serious consequences develop.

## Drug Interactions Simplified

Imagine your liver as a busy restaurant kitchen with multiple chefs (enzymes) preparing different dishes (metabolizing drugs). The cytochrome P450 (CYP450) system represents these enzyme "chefs," with each specializing in breaking down specific medications. When multiple medications need the same chef, a backup occurs—just like orders piling up when a kitchen gets too busy. This backup can cause medication levels to rise dangerously high or prevent other medications from being processed effectively.

**The "traffic jam" analogy for CYP450 interactions** helps patients understand why their antidepressant suddenly causes side effects after starting a new antibiotic. Picture a highway with multiple lanes (different CYP enzymes) where medications travel to be processed. Some medications are like slow-moving trucks that block entire lanes (enzyme inhibitors), causing traffic jams for other medications trying to use the same route. Others are like pace cars that speed up traffic flow (enzyme inducers), causing some medications to get processed too quickly (19).

For example, fluoxetine and paroxetine are notorious "lane blockers" that inhibit CYP2D6, a major enzyme processing many psychiatric medications. When a patient taking one of these SSRIs starts a beta-blocker for blood pressure, the beta-blocker can accumulate to dangerous levels because it can't get through the blocked lane. This explains why some patients suddenly develop severe fatigue or dangerously slow heart rates with medication combinations that seem unrelated (20).

**Common dangerous combinations** in psychiatric practice require heightened vigilance:

SSRIs combined with other serotonergic medications create risk for serotonin syndrome. This includes obvious combinations like two antidepressants but also hidden dangers: tramadol for pain, triptans for migraines, dextromethorphan in cough syrup, and even high-dose St. John's Wort. The risk multiplies when patients see multiple providers who don't communicate (21).

MAO inhibitors present the most serious interaction risks, requiring 14-day washout periods when switching medications and strict dietary restrictions. Despite their effectiveness, many prescribers avoid them due to interaction potential. However, understanding their mechanism—completely shutting down the enzyme that breaks down certain neurotransmitters—explains both their power and their danger (22).

Mood stabilizers interact with common medications in ways patients rarely anticipate. Lithium levels spike dangerously with NSAIDs like ibuprofen, leading to toxicity from medications patients consider harmless. Carbamazepine induces liver enzymes so powerfully it can render birth control pills ineffective, leading to unplanned pregnancies. Lamotrigine combined with valproate requires dose adjustments to prevent severe rashes (23).

## Case Example 1: The Hidden Interaction

Jennifer, a 34-year-old teacher, had taken sertraline successfully for two years. She developed a sinus infection and received antibiotics from an urgent care clinic. Within days, she experienced severe anxiety, tremors, and confusion. Her husband brought her to therapy reporting, "She's talking so fast I can't understand her, and she's sweating through her clothes."

Recognizing potential serotonin syndrome, you immediately contacted her psychiatrist while her husband drove her to the emergency department. Investigation revealed the antibiotic linezolid has MAO-inhibiting properties—information not flagged by the urgent care pharmacy system. The combination with sertraline triggered mild serotonin syndrome, resolved with medication discontinuation and supportive care.

This case highlights how interactions occur even with seemingly unrelated medications and why maintaining updated medication lists across all providers proves critical.

**Using interaction checkers effectively** requires understanding their limitations. While electronic databases flag many interactions, they often overwhelm users with theoretical risks while missing real-world problems. Learn to differentiate interaction severity levels: contraindicated combinations that should never occur, major interactions requiring close monitoring or dose adjustments, and minor interactions of limited clinical significance (24).

Free interaction checkers like Drugs.com or Medscape provide quick references, but they require clinical judgment to interpret. A checker might flag every SSRI-NSAID combination as risky, but the actual danger varies greatly between occasional ibuprofen use versus daily high-dose NSAIDs. Focus on interactions causing functional impairment or safety risks rather than every theoretical concern.

## Special Populations Overview

Certain groups face unique medication risks requiring modified approaches and extra vigilance. Understanding these vulnerabilities helps you advocate for appropriate treatment while recognizing when standard protocols need adjustment.

**Children and adolescents: Growing brains** process medications differently than adult brains, with less predictable responses and higher risks for certain adverse effects. The developing prefrontal cortex makes young people more susceptible to activation and behavioral disinhibition from antidepressants. This explains the FDA black box warning about increased suicidal ideation in youth taking antidepressants—not because medications cause suicidal thoughts directly, but because they can increase energy and impulsivity before improving mood (25).

Young people also metabolize medications faster due to efficient liver function, often requiring higher weight-based doses than adults. However, their developing brains show increased sensitivity to side effects, creating a challenging balance. Antipsychotics cause weight gain and metabolic changes more rapidly in youth, with some adolescents gaining 20-30 pounds within months. Stimulants for ADHD can significantly impact growth patterns, requiring regular monitoring of height and weight trajectories (26).

## Case Example 2: The Activated Adolescent

Fifteen-year-old Marcus started fluoxetine for depression and anxiety. Two weeks later, his mother called between sessions: "He's not himself—he's up all night rearranging his room, talking nonstop, and got in three fights at school this week. He's never been aggressive before."

Recognizing antidepressant-induced activation, you facilitated immediate psychiatric consultation. The prescriber discontinued fluoxetine and started a low-dose mood stabilizer, ultimately diagnosing bipolar disorder that the antidepressant had unmasked. Your quick recognition of activation versus normal adolescent behavior prevented potential violence and school expulsion.

**Pregnancy and breastfeeding: Two patients, one medication** creates complex risk-benefit calculations. Every medication decision affects both mother and baby, with different considerations for each trimester and postpartum period. First-trimester exposure raises concerns about organ malformation, while third-trimester exposure can cause neonatal adaptation syndromes. Breastfeeding introduces additional complexity as medications transfer through breast milk at varying concentrations (27).

The key lies in realistic risk communication. Untreated maternal mental illness carries its own risks: prenatal depression associates with preterm birth and low birth weight, while untreated bipolar disorder increases risk for poor prenatal care and substance use. Most women with moderate to severe mental illness benefit from continued treatment during pregnancy, with medication adjustments rather than discontinuation (28).

**Elderly: Start low, go slow** reflects the profound changes aging brings to medication processing. Decreased kidney and liver function means medications clear more slowly, accumulating to higher levels. Reduced muscle mass and increased fat percentage alter drug distribution. Brain changes increase sensitivity to cognitive effects, with benzodiazepines and anticholinergics causing confusion at doses well-tolerated by younger adults (29).

Polypharmacy compounds these risks as elderly patients often take multiple medications for various conditions. Each additional medication exponentially increases interaction risks. The Beers Criteria identifies potentially inappropriate medications for older adults, but clinical judgment must consider quality of life alongside safety. An elderly patient might accept increased fall risk from a benzodiazepine if it allows them to leave their house without panic attacks (30).

**Medical comorbidities: When the body changes the rules** significantly impact psychiatric medication safety. Kidney disease affects lithium clearance, requiring dose reductions and frequent monitoring. Liver disease impairs metabolism of most psychiatric medications, necessitating lower doses and longer titration periods. Cardiac conditions create vulnerability to QT prolongation from antipsychotics and certain antidepressants, potentially triggering fatal arrhythmias (31).

Less obvious comorbidities also matter. Diabetes alters medication response and increases vulnerability to metabolic side effects from antipsychotics. Thyroid disorders can mimic or exacerbate psychiatric symptoms while affecting medication metabolism. Even smoking status matters—cigarette smoke induces CYP1A2, requiring higher doses of medications like clozapine and olanzapine in smokers (32).

## Emergency Situations

Psychiatric medication emergencies require rapid recognition and decisive action. While rare, these situations can be life-threatening without prompt intervention. Your role involves recognizing warning signs, facilitating emergency care, and providing clear information to emergency responders.

**Serotonin syndrome: Too much of a good thing** occurs when excessive serotonin activity overwhelms the nervous system. Picture serotonin receptors like volume controls on a stereo—normally set at comfortable levels. Serotonin syndrome cranks every dial to maximum simultaneously, creating a cacophony of overstimulation affecting multiple body systems (33).

The syndrome presents with a triad of symptoms: mental status changes (confusion, agitation, hallucinations), autonomic dysfunction (fever, sweating, rapid heart rate, blood pressure fluctuations), and neuromuscular abnormalities (tremor, muscle rigidity, hyperreflexia). Onset typically occurs within hours to days of medication changes, distinguishing it from gradual side effect development (34).

Mild cases might present subtly—a patient seeming "jittery" with slight tremor and anxiety after adding trazodone to their SSRI. Severe cases create medical emergencies with high fever, seizures, and kidney failure. The key lies in recognizing the constellation of symptoms rather than waiting for dramatic presentations (35).

### Case Example 3: The Dangerous Supplement

David, a 45-year-old engineer, took venlafaxine for depression. Frustrated with persistent fatigue, he started multiple supplements from a health food store. During therapy, you noticed unusual symptoms: profuse sweating despite cool weather, tremulous hands making note-taking difficult, and rapid speech with mild confusion.

Questioning revealed his supplement regimen included 5-HTP, SAM-e, and high-dose St. John's Wort—all serotonergic substances. Combined with venlafaxine, they triggered moderate serotonin syndrome. Your immediate recognition led to emergency department evaluation, medication discontinuation, and full recovery within 48 hours. Without intervention, progression to severe syndrome could have caused seizures or worse.

**NMS: When antipsychotics backfire** represents a rare but potentially fatal reaction to dopamine-blocking medications. Unlike serotonin syndrome's overstimulation, NMS reflects a sudden, severe dopamine deficiency causing whole-body dysfunction. Think of dopamine as oil in an engine—blocking it too completely causes the entire system to seize up (36).

NMS develops over days to weeks with four cardinal features: hyperthermia (often exceeding 104°F), severe muscle rigidity (described as "lead pipe"), altered mental status, and autonomic instability. Laboratory findings include extremely elevated creatine kinase from muscle breakdown, which can lead to kidney failure. Mortality reaches 10-20% without prompt treatment (37).

Risk factors include high-potency antipsychotics, rapid dose increases, depot injections, and dehydration. Young males show higher susceptibility, as do patients with previous NMS episodes or organic brain conditions. Sometimes NMS occurs with antiemetics like metoclopramide that patients don't recognize as dopamine blockers (38).

**Lithium toxicity: The narrow window** demonstrates why some effective medications require careful monitoring. Lithium's therapeutic window sits precariously between ineffective and toxic levels, like walking a tightrope where small missteps cause major problems. Therapeutic levels range from 0.6-1.2 mEq/L, with toxicity beginning around 1.5 mEq/L—a dangerously narrow margin (39).

Acute toxicity typically results from overdose, while chronic toxicity develops insidiously from dehydration, drug interactions, or kidney function decline. Early symptoms include nausea, tremor, and confusion—easily mistaken for common side effects. Progressive toxicity causes severe neurological symptoms: ataxia, seizures, and coma. Permanent neurological damage can occur even with treatment (40).

Dehydration from exercise, illness, or hot weather concentrates lithium dangerously. NSAIDs reduce lithium excretion, while thiazide diuretics increase reabsorption. Even dietary sodium changes affect lithium levels—patients starting low-sodium diets can develop toxicity without dose changes (41).

## Clinical Vignette: Recognizing Serotonin Syndrome in the Therapy Office

Rebecca, a 38-year-old marketing director, arrived for her usual Wednesday afternoon therapy appointment looking visibly different. Normally composed and professionally dressed, she appeared disheveled with sweat stains despite the cool autumn weather. As she sat down, you noticed her hands trembling more than the mild caffeine-induced tremor she occasionally displayed.

"I feel so strange," she began, speaking more rapidly than usual. "I can't stop sweating, and my heart feels like it's racing. Maybe I'm getting sick?" She removed her blazer, revealing arms covered in goosebumps despite her complaint of feeling hot.

Your clinical instincts activated. Rebecca had been stable on escitalopram for six months. During check-in, she mentioned her psychiatrist added buspirone two weeks ago for residual anxiety. "Any other medication changes?" you inquired.

"Well, I saw my neurologist Monday for migraines. She gave me something new—suma-something? I took it yesterday when I felt a headache starting."

The pieces clicked together: SSRI plus buspirone plus sumatriptan—a serotonergic triple threat. You observed her closely while asking targeted questions. Her pupils appeared dilated, she shifted restlessly in her chair, and when she reached for her water bottle, her hand movements seemed jerky and uncoordinated.

"Rebecca, I'm concerned you might be experiencing a medication interaction. Let's check a few things." Using simple clinical assessments, you noted hyperreflexia when checking her knee reflex with a reflex hammer kept for such situations. Her heart rate measured 118 on the pulse oximeter—well above her usual 70s.

You explained calmly but clearly: "Your medications might be causing too much serotonin activity in your system. This is treatable, but we need to get you medical attention now." You called her psychiatrist while Rebecca contacted her husband to drive her to the emergency department, providing a written summary of medications and symptoms for the emergency team.

The emergency department confirmed mild serotonin syndrome. They discontinued medications, provided IV fluids and supportive care, and monitored her overnight. Rebecca recovered fully within 48 hours. Her psychiatrist later adjusted her regimen, and her neurologist switched to a non-serotonergic migraine medication.

Reflecting later, Rebecca expressed gratitude: "I would have gone home thinking I had the flu. You possibly saved my life by recognizing what was happening."

## Quick Reference Box: Emergency Contact Protocols

### Immediate Emergency Department Referral:

- Temperature above 101°F with psychiatric medication changes
- Severe confusion or hallucinations with physical symptoms
- Muscle rigidity with altered mental status
- Seizures or loss of consciousness
- Heart rate above 120 or below 50 with symptoms
- Blood pressure above 180/110 or below 90/60 with symptoms

**Urgent Prescriber Contact (Same Day):**

- New tremor, restlessness, or agitation after medication changes
- Significant confusion or cognitive changes
- Persistent vomiting or severe nausea
- New rash, especially with mucosal involvement
- Dizziness with falls or near-falls

**Next Business Day Contact:**

- Mild side effects affecting function
- Questions about drug interactions
- Need for dose adjustment discussions
- Medication adherence concerns

**Information to Provide:**

1. Current medications with doses and recent changes
2. Vital signs if available
3. Specific symptoms with onset timing
4. Relevant medical history
5. Contact information for follow-up

**Documentation Requirements:**

- Time and date of symptom recognition
- Actions taken and rationale
- Patient response and disposition
- Communications with providers
- Follow-up plans

## Staying Vigilant

Safety in psychopharmacology requires constant awareness without creating paralyzing anxiety. Most patients take psychiatric medications without serious adverse events, but vigilance catches problems early when intervention matters most. Your role as a frontline observer—combined with knowledge of risk factors, warning signs, and appropriate responses—creates a safety net protecting patients from preventable harm.

Understanding drug interactions, recognizing vulnerable populations, and responding effectively to emergencies transforms you from passive observer to active participant in medication safety. This knowledge empowers confident clinical practice while ensuring patients receive both effective treatment and vigilant protection from adverse events.

## Key Takeaways

- Drug interactions often occur through CYP450 enzyme competition, causing medications to accumulate or fail
- Common dangerous combinations include multiple serotonergic drugs, MAO inhibitors with many medications, and mood stabilizers with everyday drugs like NSAIDs
- Special populations—children, elderly, pregnant women, and those with medical conditions—require modified medication approaches and extra monitoring
- Serotonin syndrome presents with mental changes, autonomic dysfunction, and neuromuscular symptoms requiring immediate intervention
- NMS causes severe rigidity, high fever, and altered consciousness from antipsychotic medications
- Lithium's narrow therapeutic window makes toxicity risk constant, especially with dehydration or drug interactions
- Clear emergency protocols and prescriber communication systems prevent adverse events from becoming tragedies
- Your frequent patient contact positions you to catch safety concerns before they escalate

# Chapter 4: Antidepressants - Lifting the Fog

Depression affects one in five people during their lifetime, yet finding the right antidepressant often feels like solving a complex puzzle with missing pieces. Each medication works slightly differently, affecting unique brain pathways and producing distinct side effects. Understanding these differences transforms the frustrating trial-and-error process into informed decision-making that gets patients better faster.

## SSRIs: The First-Line Warriors

Selective serotonin reuptake inhibitors revolutionized depression treatment by offering effectiveness with fewer side effects than older medications. Think of SSRIs as precision tools rather than sledgehammers—they target specific brain chemistry without affecting multiple systems simultaneously.

**How They Work: The serotonin "drain plug" mechanism** functions exactly as the name suggests. After serotonin delivers its mood-regulating message across the synapse, the sending brain cell normally vacuums it back up for recycling. SSRIs block this vacuum system, like putting a plug in a drain. The serotonin stays in the synapse longer, continuing to activate mood-improving signals. This elegant mechanism explains why SSRIs help depression, anxiety, and obsessive-compulsive symptoms—all conditions involving serotonin signaling problems (42).

**The Big Six** SSRIs each have unique properties despite sharing the same basic mechanism. Understanding these differences helps match the right medication to each patient's specific needs.

**Fluoxetine (Prozac)** stands out for its long half-life of 4-6 days, meaning it leaves the body slowly. This provides built-in protection against withdrawal symptoms if patients miss doses, but also means side effects linger longer. Starting doses typically range from 10-20 mg daily, increasing to 40-60 mg for full effect. The activating properties help patients with low energy but might worsen anxiety initially (43).

**Sertraline (Zoloft)** offers a middle ground with moderate half-life and balanced effects. Starting at 25-50 mg daily and increasing to 100-200 mg, it causes fewer drug interactions than fluoxetine. Many clinicians favor sertraline as a first choice due to its effectiveness across depression and anxiety disorders with manageable side effects (44).

**Paroxetine (Paxil)** provides strong anti-anxiety effects but causes more side effects than other SSRIs. Its short half-life leads to withdrawal symptoms if doses are missed. Starting doses of 10-20 mg increase to 40-60 mg daily. Weight gain and sexual dysfunction occur more frequently with paroxetine, making it less popular despite its effectiveness (45).

**Citalopram (Celexa)** and **escitalopram (Lexapro)** are chemical cousins, with escitalopram being a refined version of citalopram. Escitalopram typically works at half the dose—10 mg of escitalopram equals roughly 20 mg of citalopram. Both cause minimal drug interactions. However, citalopram carries dose restrictions due to heart rhythm concerns at higher doses (46).

**Fluvoxamine (Luvox)**, primarily used for obsessive-compulsive disorder, requires twice-daily dosing and causes significant drug interactions. Its use remains limited despite effectiveness for anxiety disorders (47).

**Dosing strategies and titration** follow the principle of "start low, go slow" to minimize side effects while achieving therapeutic benefits. Most patients start at half the target dose for one to two weeks before increasing. This gradual approach allows the brain to adjust, reducing nausea, headaches, and anxiety that commonly occur initially.

**Side effect profiles and management** vary among SSRIs but share common themes. Gastrointestinal upset affects 20-30% of patients initially but usually resolves within two weeks. Taking medication with food helps. Sexual dysfunction—decreased libido, delayed orgasm, or erectile dysfunction—affects up to 70% of patients and persists throughout treatment. Strategies include dose reduction, drug holidays, or adding medications like bupropion to counteract these effects (48).

Sleep changes occur bidirectionally. Some patients experience drowsiness (particularly with paroxetine), while others develop insomnia (especially with fluoxetine). Timing doses accordingly—morning for activating effects, evening for sedating ones—often resolves sleep issues without additional medications.

**Clinical Pearls** for SSRI management come from years of practical experience. **Morning vs. evening dosing** depends on individual response rather than medication choice. Start with morning dosing, then adjust based on patient experience. If insomnia develops, try evening dosing. If daytime drowsiness occurs, return to morning administration.

**Sexual side effects** represent the elephant in the room—everyone knows they're common, but nobody wants to discuss them. Normalize the conversation by bringing it up proactively: "Many people experience changes in sexual function with these medications. It's nothing to be embarrassed about, and we have strategies to help if it becomes a problem." Document sexual function before starting SSRIs to establish baseline. Consider medications with lower sexual side effect rates (like bupropion) for sexually active patients when appropriate (49).

**Withdrawal symptoms** catch patients off-guard when they stop SSRIs abruptly. "Brain zaps," dizziness, flu-like symptoms, and mood changes can occur, particularly with short-acting medications like paroxetine. Planning ahead prevents problems—taper over 2-4 weeks minimum, longer for medications taken over a year. Create written taper schedules and warn patients about potential symptoms to prevent panic if they occur (50).

## Case Vignette: John's Journey from Lexapro to Zoloft

John, a 35-year-old accountant, started escitalopram 10 mg for depression and generalized anxiety. After six weeks, his mood improved significantly, but he developed problems that threatened his marriage. "I feel better emotionally," he explained, "but I have zero interest in sex. My wife thinks I'm not attracted to her anymore."

Despite trying various strategies—dose reduction to 5 mg, weekend drug holidays, timing changes—the sexual dysfunction persisted. His psychiatrist suggested switching to sertraline, which sometimes causes fewer sexual side effects. The transition required careful planning to prevent withdrawal symptoms and mood destabilization.

Week 1: Reduced escitalopram to 5 mg while adding sertraline 25 mg Week 2: Stopped escitalopram, increased sertraline to 50 mg Week 3-4: Gradually increased sertraline to 100 mg

John experienced mild dizziness during the switch but no significant mood changes. After eight weeks on sertraline 100 mg, his depression remained controlled with notably improved sexual function. "It's not perfect," he reported, "but it's good enough that my marriage is back on track."

This case illustrates how individual responses to SSRIs vary dramatically and switching within the class can resolve intolerable side effects while maintaining therapeutic benefits.

## SNRIs: The Dual-Action Approach

Serotonin-norepinephrine reuptake inhibitors add a second mechanism to the SSRI model, simultaneously targeting mood and energy pathways. This dual action provides advantages for specific patient populations but also introduces additional considerations.

**Mechanism: Closing two drains instead of one** means SNRIs block reuptake of both serotonin and norepinephrine. Think of it as plugging two drains in connected sinks—both neurotransmitter levels rise, affecting mood through serotonin and energy/focus through norepinephrine. This combination particularly benefits patients with depression featuring prominent fatigue, poor concentration, or physical pain symptoms (51).

**When to Choose SNRIs** depends on symptom profiles and previous medication responses. **Depression with pain** responds particularly well to SNRIs. The norepinephrine effects modulate pain signals in the spinal cord, explaining why these medications help fibromyalgia, neuropathy, and chronic pain syndromes. Patients often report both mood improvement and pain reduction—a double benefit impossible with SSRIs alone (52).

**Energy and motivation issues** that don't respond to SSRIs might improve with SNRIs. The norepinephrine boost acts like a gentle stimulant, improving focus and drive without the risks of actual stimulants. This makes SNRIs valuable for depression with prominent cognitive symptoms or when patients can't tolerate traditional stimulants.

**Venlafaxine (Effexor)** demonstrates dose-dependent effects. At doses below 150 mg, it acts mainly as an SSRI. Norepinephrine effects emerge at higher doses, allowing customization based on patient needs. Extended-release formulations reduce side effects and allow once-daily dosing. Maximum doses reach 375 mg daily for severe depression (53).

**Duloxetine (Cymbalta)** affects both neurotransmitters at all doses, starting at 30 mg daily and increasing to 60-120 mg. FDA approval for multiple pain conditions makes it a logical choice when depression coexists with chronic pain. The capsule formulation can't be split, limiting dosing flexibility (54).

**Desvenlafaxine (Pristiq)**, the active metabolite of venlafaxine, offers similar effects with potentially fewer drug interactions. The 50 mg starting dose is also the therapeutic dose for many patients, simplifying titration. However, higher doses don't necessarily increase effectiveness and may worsen side effects (55).

**Managing Blood Pressure: The norepinephrine effect** creates unique monitoring needs. Norepinephrine increases heart rate and blood pressure, particularly at higher doses. While usually mild, these effects can be significant in patients with hypertension or cardiac disease. Regular blood pressure monitoring during dose increases helps identify problems early. Most patients tolerate these effects, but some require antihypertensive adjustment or medication switching (56).

**Clinical Pearl: Venlafaxine withdrawal - why it's different** stems from its short half-life combined with dual neurotransmitter effects. Missing even one dose can trigger severe withdrawal symptoms— "brain zaps," vertigo, nausea, and mood swings—within hours. Patients describe feeling like they have severe flu combined with electrical shocks in their brain. Prevention requires meticulous adherence and extremely gradual tapering over months, not weeks. Consider switching to fluoxetine before tapering to leverage its long half-life for smoother discontinuation (57).

## Atypical Antidepressants: The Specialists

When standard antidepressants fail or cause intolerable side effects, atypical options offer unique mechanisms and side effect profiles. These medications work through diverse pathways, providing solutions for specific clinical challenges.

**Bupropion: The activating option** stands apart by affecting dopamine and norepinephrine without touching serotonin. This unique mechanism produces a stimulant-like effect without controlled substance risks. Starting at 150 mg daily and increasing to 300-450 mg, bupropion requires divided dosing in immediate-release form or once-daily administration with extended-release versions (58).

**No sexual side effects** makes bupropion invaluable for sexually active patients. Rather than causing dysfunction, it might actually improve libido and sexual response. This property leads to its use as an add-on medication to counteract SSRI-induced sexual dysfunction. Some patients take bupropion only on weekends to enhance sexual function while maintaining their primary antidepressant (59).

34

**Weight loss potential** averages 5-10 pounds, contrasting sharply with weight gain from many psychiatric medications. The appetite suppression and increased energy expenditure make bupropion helpful for patients concerned about weight, though it's not a weight loss medication per se. Patients with eating disorders require careful monitoring as weight loss can trigger relapse (60).

**Seizure risk considerations** limit bupropion use in certain populations. The risk increases with higher doses, rapid titration, eating disorders, head trauma history, or alcohol withdrawal. Maximum daily doses shouldn't exceed 450 mg, with no single dose over 200 mg for immediate-release formulations. Despite these precautions, seizures remain rare in properly selected patients (61).

**Mirtazapine: The sleep and appetite helper** works through a complex mechanism blocking specific serotonin and norepinephrine receptors while enhancing their release. Think of it as fine-tuning a radio—blocking static while amplifying the desired signal. This produces reliable improvements in sleep and appetite, often within days of starting treatment (62).

**The paradox of lower doses** confuses many clinicians. At 7.5-15 mg, mirtazapine causes significant sedation through antihistamine effects. At 30-45 mg, norepinephrine effects emerge, reducing sedation and improving energy. This means increasing the dose might actually reduce drowsiness—counterintuitive but clinically important. Start low for primary insomnia, higher for depression with insomnia (63).

**Combination strategies** using mirtazapine with SSRIs or SNRIs create powerful antidepressant effects. The combination, sometimes called "California rocket fuel," helps treatment-resistant depression by attacking multiple neurotransmitter systems simultaneously. Adding mirtazapine 15-30 mg at bedtime to an SSRI can improve sleep, appetite, and overall antidepressant response while potentially reducing SSRI-induced sexual dysfunction (64).

## Case Study: Choosing the Right Antidepressant for Maria

Maria, a 44-year-old marketing manager, presented with her third major depressive episode. Previous trials of sertraline caused intolerable fatigue despite mood improvement. Escitalopram triggered 25-pound weight gain over six months, worsening her self-esteem. She needed an antidepressant that wouldn't cause weight gain or sedation while effectively treating her depression.

Initial assessment revealed:

- Prominent symptoms: low mood, poor concentration, lack of motivation
- Minimal anxiety symptoms
- Concerned about weight and sexual function
- History of good response to SSRIs except for side effects
- No seizure risk factors
- Mild hypertension, well-controlled

Bupropion emerged as the logical choice given her specific needs. Starting at 150 mg XL each morning, she noticed improved energy within a week—earlier than typical antidepressant response. After two weeks, the dose increased to 300 mg XL daily.

Six weeks later, Maria reported significant improvement: "I feel like myself again, but better. I've lost 8 pounds without trying, my concentration is sharp, and my husband is thrilled that my sex drive returned." Her only complaint involved mild insomnia, resolved by taking medication immediately upon waking rather than with breakfast.

At three-month follow-up, Maria remained in remission with sustained weight loss and no sexual side effects. This case demonstrates how matching medication selection to individual patient priorities and previous response patterns improves outcomes and adherence.

## Older Antidepressants: Still Relevant

While newer isn't always better, older antidepressants require more careful management due to their broader effects and higher side effect burden. Understanding when these medications shine helps serve patients who don't respond to modern options.

**TCAs: Powerful but demanding respect** work through what's called the "shotgun approach"—affecting multiple neurotransmitter systems simultaneously. Unlike the precision of SSRIs, tricyclic antidepressants impact serotonin, norepinephrine, histamine, acetylcholine, and various other receptors. This broad action explains both their effectiveness and their challenging side effect profile (65).

Common TCAs include amitriptyline, nortriptyline, imipramine, and desipramine. They share similar mechanisms but differ in potency and side effect emphasis. Tertiary amines (amitriptyline, imipramine) cause more side effects than secondary amines (nortriptyline, desipramine), making the latter preferable when TCAs are needed (66).

**Monitoring requirements** for TCAs exceed those of newer antidepressants. Baseline EKG identifies cardiac conduction abnormalities that contraindicate use. Blood levels help optimize dosing—too low proves ineffective while too high risks toxicity. Therapeutic drug monitoring particularly helps with nortriptyline, which has a well-defined therapeutic window of 50-150 ng/mL (67).

Side effects follow predictable patterns based on receptor blockade:

- Anticholinergic: dry mouth, constipation, urinary retention, blurred vision
- Antihistamine: sedation, weight gain
- Alpha-blocking: orthostatic hypotension, dizziness
- Cardiac: conduction delays, arrhythmia risk in overdose

**Clinical Pearl: Using TCAs for chronic pain** leverages their broad receptor effects beneficially. Low doses (10-50 mg) of amitriptyline or nortriptyline effectively treat neuropathic pain, fibromyalgia, and migraine prevention—often at doses below antidepressant levels. The pain relief occurs independently of mood effects, helping even nondepressed patients. Starting with 10 mg at bedtime and increasing slowly minimizes side effects while achieving pain control (68).

**MAOIs: The last resort that sometimes works best** inhibit monoamine oxidase enzymes responsible for breaking down serotonin, norepinephrine, and dopamine. By shutting down this disposal system, MAOIs create powerful antidepressant effects in patients who don't respond to other medications. However, they also break down tyramine from food, creating potential for dangerous interactions (69).

Available MAOIs include phenelzine (Nardil), tranylcypromine (Parnate), and the patch formulation selegiline (Emsam). The patch bypasses gut MAO inhibition at low doses, reducing dietary restrictions. Higher doses require full dietary precautions regardless of formulation (70).

**Dietary restrictions made simple** focus on avoiding aged, fermented, or spoiled foods high in tyramine. Fresh foods pose no risk. The restricted list includes:

- Aged cheeses (except cottage cheese, cream cheese)
- Cured or processed meats (pepperoni, salami, jerky)
- Fermented foods (sauerkraut, soy sauce, miso)
- Draft beer and red wine
- Overripe bananas
- Broad bean pods

Fresh meat, poultry, fish, and most fruits and vegetables remain safe. Restaurant eating requires caution but remains possible with education. Many patients successfully follow these restrictions for years when MAOIs provide relief unavailable from other medications (71).

## Moving Forward with Antidepressant Knowledge

Understanding antidepressants requires appreciating both their similarities and crucial differences. While all ultimately improve mood, their distinct mechanisms, side effects, and clinical applications make medication selection as much art as science. The key lies in matching medication properties to individual patient needs, previous responses, and life circumstances.

Modern antidepressants offer safer, more tolerable options than previous generations, but older medications retain important roles for specific situations. By understanding each class's strengths and limitations, clinicians can guide patients through the sometimes frustrating process of finding the right medication match.

**Key Takeaways**

- SSRIs work by blocking serotonin reuptake, effectively increasing serotonin activity in mood-regulating brain circuits
- Each SSRI has unique properties regarding half-life, drug interactions, and side effect profiles that guide selection
- Sexual dysfunction affects most SSRI users but can be managed through dose adjustment, drug holidays, or medication switching
- SNRIs add norepinephrine effects to serotonin action, particularly helping depression with pain, fatigue, or cognitive symptoms
- Venlafaxine withdrawal requires extremely careful management due to severe discontinuation symptoms
- Bupropion offers unique benefits of no sexual side effects and potential weight loss but requires seizure risk screening
- Mirtazapine's sedation decreases at higher doses while antidepressant effects increase
- TCAs remain valuable for chronic pain and treatment-resistant depression despite greater side effect burden
- MAOIs can help patients who don't respond to other antidepressants but require careful dietary adherence
- Matching medication selection to individual patient priorities improves both outcomes and adherence

# Chapter 5: Mood Stabilizers - Finding Balance

Bipolar disorder affects 4% of adults during their lifetime, causing devastating mood swings that destroy relationships, careers, and lives without proper treatment. Mood stabilizers prevent these extremes, acting like shock absorbers that dampen emotional oscillations. Unlike antidepressants that lift mood in one direction, mood stabilizers maintain equilibrium—preventing both manic highs and depressive lows.

## Lithium: The Gold Standard

For over 70 years, lithium has remained psychiatry's most effective mood stabilizer despite being a simple salt. Its discovery revolutionized bipolar treatment, transforming a usually fatal illness into a manageable condition. Understanding lithium's unique properties, requirements, and risks helps clinicians support patients through successful long-term treatment.

**Mechanism: Stabilizing the cell's electrical system** involves multiple complex actions simplified into practical understanding. Think of brain cells as having electrical systems like a house. During mood episodes, these systems malfunction—mania resembles electrical surges while depression mirrors power failures. Lithium acts like a whole-house surge protector and voltage regulator, preventing extremes in either direction (72).

At the cellular level, lithium affects second messenger systems, particularly those involving inositol and protein kinase C. These pathways regulate how cells respond to neurotransmitter signals. By modulating these systems, lithium prevents excessive responses without blocking normal function—maintaining mood stability without emotional blunting (73).

**The Therapeutic Window** for lithium remains remarkably narrow, requiring careful monitoring to balance effectiveness with safety. Therapeutic levels typically range from 0.6-1.2 mEq/L for maintenance, with acute mania sometimes requiring temporary increases to 0.8-1.5 mEq/L. The challenge lies in this tight range—below 0.6 often proves ineffective while above 1.5 risks toxicity (74).

**Understanding blood levels** requires appreciating multiple factors affecting lithium concentration:

- Timing matters: levels must be drawn 12 hours after the last dose for accuracy
- Steady state takes 5-7 days after dose changes
- Kidney function directly impacts lithium clearance
- Dehydration concentrates lithium dangerously
- Drug interactions alter lithium levels unpredictably

**Monitoring schedule simplified** follows a practical pattern. Initially, check levels weekly until stable, then monthly for three months, then every 3-6 months indefinitely. Also monitor kidney function (creatinine) and thyroid (TSH) every 6-12 months since lithium affects both organs long-term. This might seem excessive, but catching problems early prevents serious complications (75).

**Managing Side Effects** requires understanding lithium's impact on multiple body systems. The **"three Ps": Polyuria, polydipsia, and practical solutions** describe lithium's effect on kidney concentrating ability. Patients urinate frequently (polyuria) and drink excessively (polydipsia) as kidneys lose ability to concentrate urine. This proves more than inconvenient—it disrupts sleep, work, and social activities.

Practical solutions include:

- Taking lithium at bedtime to minimize daytime urination
- Using controlled-release formulations
- Avoiding caffeine and alcohol which worsen symptoms
- Considering once-daily dosing if tolerated
- Adding amiloride if symptoms severely impact quality of life

**Tremor management strategies** address another common side effect affecting 25-50% of lithium users. This fine, rapid hand tremor differs from parkinsonian tremor, worsening with intentional movement. Strategies include:

41

- Reducing caffeine intake
- Dividing doses or using extended-release formulations
- Adding propranolol 10-40 mg for significant tremor
- Ensuring levels remain in lower therapeutic range
- Evaluating thyroid function since hypothyroidism worsens tremor

**Clinical Pearls** from decades of lithium use guide practical management. **Dehydration dangers** top the safety list. Any condition causing fluid loss—fever, vomiting, diarrhea, excessive sweating—concentrates lithium potentially to toxic levels. Patients need clear instructions: "If you get sick and can't keep fluids down, stop lithium temporarily and contact your prescriber." Summer heat, intense exercise, and low-sodium diets all require extra vigilance (76).

**NSAIDs and lithium don't mix** represents a critical drug interaction often overlooked. Ibuprofen, naproxen, and other NSAIDs reduce kidney lithium clearance, potentially doubling blood levels within days. While aspirin and acetaminophen remain safe, many patients don't realize common pain relievers can cause lithium toxicity. Education prevents emergency situations: "Always check with your pharmacist before taking over-the-counter pain medications" (77).

**Lithium monitoring schedule** deserves prominent display in every clinical setting:

- Baseline: CBC, electrolytes, creatinine, TSH, EKG if over 50
- Week 1 and weekly until stable: lithium level
- Months 1-3: monthly lithium level, creatinine
- Months 3-6: lithium level every 3 months
- Long-term: lithium level, creatinine, TSH every 6 months
- Any dose change: level after 5-7 days
- Suspected toxicity: immediate level, electrolytes, creatinine

## Case Vignette: Sarah's Lithium Success Story

Sarah, a 28-year-old graduate student, experienced her second manic episode after stopping medication believing she was "cured." The first episode two years prior led to hospitalization after she spent $15,000 on craft supplies for a business she impulsively started, went five days without sleep, and believed she could communicate telepathically with her professors.

Starting lithium proved challenging. Initial dosing at 300 mg twice daily produced levels of only 0.4 mEq/L—subtherapeutic. Increasing to 450 mg twice daily achieved 0.7 mEq/L, but Sarah complained of excessive urination disrupting her classes. Switching to 900 mg of extended-release lithium at bedtime maintained therapeutic levels while reducing daytime urination.

Three months later, Sarah developed hand tremor affecting her laboratory work. Rather than discontinuing lithium, her psychiatrist added propranolol 20 mg twice daily, resolving the tremor without compromising mood stability. Thyroid monitoring revealed subclinical hypothyroidism (TSH 5.8), treated with levothyroxine.

Education proved critical when Sarah developed gastroenteritis six months later. Remembering warnings about dehydration, she temporarily stopped lithium and maintained hydration with electrolyte solutions. Levels checked after recovery showed no toxicity.

Two years later, Sarah remains stable on lithium with no mood episodes. She manages side effects effectively, understanding that minor inconveniences pale compared to mania's devastation. "Lithium gave me my life back," she reflects. "The monitoring and side effects are just part of staying well."

## Anticonvulsants as Mood Stabilizers

Originally developed for epilepsy, several anticonvulsants effectively prevent mood episodes through mechanisms distinct from lithium. These medications offer alternatives for patients who can't tolerate or don't respond to lithium, each with unique benefits and challenges.

**Valproic Acid: The multipurpose medication** works by enhancing GABA activity and affecting multiple cellular signaling pathways.

Available as valproate, divalproex, and extended-release formulations, they're essentially the same medication in different forms. Therapeutic levels range from 50-125 µg/mL, though some patients respond outside this range (78).

**Teratogenicity concerns** make valproic acid particularly dangerous during pregnancy. Neural tube defects occur in 1-2% of exposed fetuses, with risk highest during the first trimester. Additionally, in utero exposure associates with lower IQ and increased autism risk. Women of childbearing potential require reliable contraception and careful counseling about pregnancy risks. Many experts avoid valproic acid entirely in women who might become pregnant (79).

**Weight gain management** challenges many patients on valproic acid, with average gains of 10-20 pounds common. The mechanism involves increased appetite, altered metabolism, and insulin resistance. Strategies include:

- Baseline weight and metabolic monitoring
- Dietary counseling before weight gain occurs
- Regular exercise programs
- Considering metformin for significant weight gain
- Switching medications if weight gain threatens health or adherence

**Lab monitoring essentials** include checking levels 5 days after dose changes, then every 3-6 months when stable. Also monitor CBC (thrombocytopenia risk), liver function (hepatotoxicity), and ammonia levels if mental status changes occur. Women require regular pregnancy testing. Though monitoring seems burdensome, it catches problems before they become serious (80).

**Lamotrigine: The depression fighter** stands unique among mood stabilizers for preventing depressive episodes more than manic ones. Its mechanism involves blocking voltage-gated sodium channels and modulating glutamate release. Unlike other mood stabilizers, lamotrigine doesn't cause weight gain or sedation, improving adherence (81).

**The critical slow titration** prevents Stevens-Johnson syndrome, a potentially fatal rash. Standard titration starts at 25 mg daily for two weeks, then 50 mg for two weeks, increasing by 50 mg every two weeks to target dose of 200 mg. Valproic acid doubles lamotrigine levels, requiring even slower titration starting at 25 mg every other day. This snail's pace frustrates patients wanting quick relief but prevents devastating complications (82).

**Rash recognition and prevention** requires vigilant monitoring during titration. Any rash demands immediate evaluation, though most prove benign. Danger signs include:

- Rash with fever or flu-like symptoms
- Mucosal involvement (mouth, eyes, genitals)
- Facial swelling
- Widespread or rapidly spreading rash
- Any rash in the first 8 weeks of treatment

**Clinical Pearl: Why patience prevents Stevens-Johnson** relates to immune system sensitization. Rapid dose increases overwhelm immune tolerance, triggering severe reactions. The slow titration allows gradual accommodation. Patients who previously developed rash with rapid titration sometimes tolerate reintroduction with ultra-slow increases. Education helps: "Think of it like slowly entering a hot bath—jump in too fast and you'll get burned" (83).

**Carbamazepine: The enzyme inducer** effectively prevents mood episodes but creates complex management challenges. By powerfully inducing liver enzymes, particularly CYP3A4, carbamazepine speeds metabolism of numerous medications including birth control pills, making them ineffective. This property also causes auto-induction—carbamazepine speeds its own metabolism, requiring dose increases over time (84).

**Drug interaction complexity** makes carbamazepine challenging in patients taking multiple medications. Common problematic interactions include:

- Oral contraceptives: use alternative birth control

45

- Warfarin: requires close INR monitoring
- Other psychiatric medications: levels may drop significantly
- HIV medications: often contraindicated
- Direct oral anticoagulants: effectiveness reduced

**When it's the right choice** depends on specific clinical scenarios. Carbamazepine excels for:

- Rapid cycling bipolar disorder
- Mixed episodes with prominent irritability
- Patients who failed lithium and valproic acid
- Those requiring anti-aggression effects
- Trigeminal neuralgia comorbidity

Despite challenges, some patients respond uniquely well to carbamazepine when other mood stabilizers fail (85).

## Case Study: Transitioning from Lithium to Lamotrigine

Marcus, a 38-year-old chef, developed progressive kidney dysfunction after 10 years on lithium. His creatinine rose from 1.0 to 1.8 mg/dL, indicating significant impairment. Despite excellent mood control on lithium, continuing risked dialysis within years. The challenge: transitioning to alternative mood stabilization without triggering relapse.

Initial assessment revealed:

- Predominantly depressive episodes between rare hypomanic periods
- Lithium level 0.8 mEq/L providing good control
- Mild cognitive complaints possibly from lithium
- No history of severe mania or psychosis
- Strong preference to avoid weight gain

Lamotrigine emerged as the logical choice given his depressive pattern and need for weight-neutral options. The transition required careful orchestration:

Weeks 1-2: Started lamotrigine 25 mg daily while maintaining lithium
Weeks 3-4: Increased lamotrigine to 50 mg, reduced lithium by 25%
Weeks 5-6: Lamotrigine 100 mg, lithium reduced by 50% Weeks 7-8:
Lamotrigine 150 mg, lithium reduced by 75% Weeks 9-10:
Lamotrigine 200 mg, discontinued lithium

Throughout the transition, Marcus maintained mood stability with
mild anxiety during lithium reductions. His kidney function began
improving within months of stopping lithium. One year later, he
remained stable on lamotrigine 200 mg with creatinine improved to
1.3 mg/dL.

"The slow switch felt endless," Marcus reflected, "but my thinking is
clearer and I don't miss the constant bathroom trips. Most importantly,
my kidneys are recovering."

## Combination Strategies

Real-world bipolar disorder often requires multiple mood stabilizers
for adequate control. Understanding rational combinations improves
outcomes while minimizing risks and side effects.

**When one isn't enough** becomes apparent through persistent
breakthrough episodes despite therapeutic levels and good adherence.
Rather than abandoning partially effective medications, adding
complementary agents often achieves full stabilization. Signs
suggesting combination therapy include:

- Partial response leaving subsyndromal symptoms
- Different medications controlling different poles (mania vs.
  depression)
- Inability to reach therapeutic doses due to side effects
- Rapid cycling requiring multiple mechanisms

**Common combinations and rationales** follow evidence-based
patterns. Lithium plus lamotrigine combines lithium's antimanic
properties with lamotrigine's antidepressant effects—ideal for patients
experiencing both poles. Lithium plus valproic acid provides "double

coverage" for severe or psychotic mania, though monitoring becomes complex. Lamotrigine plus antipsychotics help when depression predominates but psychotic features require dopamine blockade (86).

Adding antipsychotics to mood stabilizers represents a frequent strategy. Quetiapine, aripiprazole, and lurasidone have specific FDA approvals for bipolar depression. Olanzapine and risperidone excel for acute mania and maintenance. These combinations often succeed when mood stabilizers alone fail (87).

**Monitoring multiple mood stabilizers** multiplies complexity exponentially. Each medication requires its own monitoring schedule, and interactions between them demand extra vigilance. Create comprehensive monitoring calendars including:

- Individual drug level requirements
- Overlapping laboratory needs (combine draws when possible)
- Drug interaction checks with each change
- Side effect assessment tools
- Clear documentation systems

Patient education becomes even more critical with combinations. Provide written schedules, use smartphone reminders, and ensure patients understand why each medication matters. Simplify regimens when possible—once-daily dosing improves adherence over multiple daily doses.

## Achieving Stability Through Understanding

Mood stabilizers save lives by preventing the destructive extremes of bipolar disorder. While each medication presents unique challenges, understanding their mechanisms, monitoring requirements, and management strategies transforms daunting complexity into manageable treatment plans. The goal isn't perfection but rather finding the right balance between effectiveness and tolerability for each individual patient.

48

Success requires patience from both clinicians and patients. Unlike antidepressants that might show benefits within weeks, mood stabilizers prove their worth by what doesn't happen—the absence of mood episodes over months and years. This preventive action requires faith in the process and commitment to long-term monitoring.

## Key Takeaways

- Lithium remains the gold standard mood stabilizer but requires careful monitoring due to its narrow therapeutic window
- Dehydration and NSAIDs represent major safety risks with lithium requiring patient education
- Valproic acid offers broad-spectrum mood stabilization but causes weight gain and severe teratogenicity
- Lamotrigine uniquely prevents depressive episodes but requires extremely slow titration to prevent dangerous rashes
- Carbamazepine induces liver enzymes creating complex drug interactions including oral contraceptive failure
- Combination mood stabilizer therapy often necessary for adequate control but multiplies monitoring requirements
- Success with mood stabilizers measured by prevented episodes rather than acute improvement
- Patient education about monitoring requirements and safety precautions prevents most serious complications
- Individual medication selection depends on episode pattern, side effect tolerance, and comorbid conditions
- Long-term adherence improves when patients understand both benefits and risks of their specific regimen

# Chapter 6: Antipsychotics - Beyond Psychosis

The term "antipsychotic" misleads many clinicians and patients, suggesting these medications only treat schizophrenia or acute psychosis. In reality, modern psychiatric practice uses antipsychotics for bipolar disorder, severe depression, anxiety disorders, and numerous other conditions. Understanding their mechanisms, benefits, and risks helps clinicians support the millions of patients who benefit from these powerful yet challenging medications.

## Understanding Antipsychotics

The journey from first-generation "typical" antipsychotics to modern "atypical" agents reflects psychiatry's evolving understanding of brain function and medication design. Each generation brought improvements but also new challenges requiring careful consideration.

**First vs. Second Generation: What really matters** goes beyond marketing labels to practical differences affecting patient care. First-generation antipsychotics like haloperidol and chlorpromazine powerfully block dopamine D2 receptors throughout the brain. This robust blockade effectively treats positive symptoms of psychosis—hallucinations, delusions, disorganized thinking—but causes significant movement side effects by blocking dopamine in motor circuits (88).

Second-generation antipsychotics added serotonin receptor blockade and other mechanisms to dopamine effects. This broader action reduces movement side effects while potentially improving mood and negative symptoms. However, they brought new problems: weight gain, diabetes, and lipid abnormalities. The distinction matters less than understanding each medication's specific profile (89).

**The Dopamine Story: Why blocking isn't always bad** requires understanding dopamine's multiple roles. In psychosis, excessive dopamine activity in mesolimbic pathways creates hallucinations and delusions. Blocking these receptors reduces psychotic symptoms. But dopamine also regulates movement, reward, and hormone secretion. Blocking dopamine in these areas causes side effects: movement disorders, anhedonia, and elevated prolactin (90).

The art lies in achieving sufficient mesolimbic blockade for symptom control while minimizing blockade elsewhere. Different antipsychotics achieve this balance through varying receptor binding patterns, explaining their distinct effects and side effect profiles.

**Mechanisms Simplified** helps predict medication effects. Think of **First-generation as "volume controls"** that turn down dopamine signaling throughout the brain. Like using a master volume knob, you can't selectively adjust different speakers. High-potency agents (haloperidol, fluphenazine) powerfully block D2 receptors at low doses, while low-potency agents (chlorpromazine, thioridazine) require higher doses for equivalent dopamine blockade but affect more receptor types (91).

**Second-generation as "smart mixers"** offer more nuanced control, adjusting multiple neurotransmitter systems independently. Risperidone blocks dopamine and serotonin in specific ratios. Quetiapine adds histamine and norepinephrine effects. Aripiprazole partially activates dopamine receptors rather than blocking them— like a dimmer switch versus an on/off switch. These varied mechanisms allow tailoring to specific symptoms (92).

## Clinical Uses Beyond Schizophrenia

Modern antipsychotic use extends far beyond their original indication, with compelling evidence for multiple psychiatric conditions. Understanding these applications helps clinicians consider antipsychotics appropriately while avoiding overuse.

**Bipolar Disorder: Mania and maintenance** represents the most common non-psychotic use of antipsychotics. During acute mania, antipsychotics work faster than mood stabilizers alone, often controlling agitation within hours. Olanzapine, risperidone, and aripiprazole demonstrate particular efficacy. For maintenance, several antipsychotics prevent both manic and depressive episodes, sometimes outperforming traditional mood stabilizers (93).

The mechanism extends beyond dopamine blockade. Antipsychotics affect cellular signaling pathways similar to lithium, providing mood stabilization independent of antipsychotic effects. This explains why lower doses often suffice for bipolar disorder compared to schizophrenia.

**Depression Augmentation: When antidepressants need help** addresses the 30% of depressed patients who don't respond adequately to antidepressants alone. Adding low-dose antipsychotics can break through treatment resistance. Aripiprazole, quetiapine, and olanzapine (combined with fluoxetine) have FDA approval for this indication. The combination often works within 1-2 weeks—faster than switching antidepressants (94).

Mechanisms remain incompletely understood but likely involve:

- Enhancing serotonin and norepinephrine signaling
- Modulating dopamine in reward circuits
- Affecting neuroplasticity and cellular resilience
- Improving sleep architecture

**Anxiety and OCD: Off-label but effective** uses leverage antipsychotics' broad receptor effects. Low-dose quetiapine (25-100 mg) helps severe anxiety through antihistamine and serotonin effects without significant dopamine blockade. Risperidone and aripiprazole augment SSRIs for treatment-resistant OCD, possibly by modulating serotonin-dopamine interactions in orbitofrontal circuits (95).

## Case Vignette: Using Abilify for Treatment-Resistant Depression

Janet, a 48-year-old teacher, struggled with her third antidepressant trial in two years. Sertraline initially helped but lost effectiveness. Venlafaxine caused intolerable blood pressure increases. Currently on duloxetine 60 mg for four months, she reported: "It's better than nothing, but I'm still barely functioning. I cry driving to work, can't concentrate on lesson plans, and spend weekends in bed."

Her psychiatrist suggested adding aripiprazole, explaining: "Sometimes antidepressants need a boost. Abilify works differently, helping your current medication work better." Janet expressed concern: "Isn't that for schizophrenia? I'm not psychotic."

Education addressed her fears: "Abilify helps many conditions at different doses. For depression, we use 2-10 mg—much lower than for psychosis. Think of it like aspirin—low doses prevent heart attacks while high doses treat pain. Same medication, different purposes."

Starting at 2 mg daily, Janet noticed improvement within 10 days: "The fog started lifting. I could think clearly again." After increasing to 5 mg, she achieved remission within a month. Side effects remained minimal—mild restlessness resolved by taking medication at bedtime.

Eight months later, Janet continues combination therapy with sustained remission. "I was terrified of taking an 'antipsychotic,' but it gave me my life back. I wish I'd tried it sooner instead of suffering through failed antidepressants."

## Managing Metabolic Effects

The metabolic consequences of antipsychotics represent their most serious long-term risks, potentially shortening lifespan through diabetes and cardiovascular disease. Understanding and managing these effects protects patients while maintaining psychiatric stability.

**The Weight Gain Hierarchy: Which drugs cause most gain** follows predictable patterns. Clozapine and olanzapine cause the most severe weight gain—often 20-30 pounds or more. Quetiapine and risperidone cause moderate gain. Aripiprazole, ziprasidone, and lurasidone remain relatively weight-neutral. Individual responses vary, but these patterns guide initial selection (96).

Weight gain mechanisms involve:

- Increased appetite through histamine and serotonin blockade
- Altered leptin and ghrelin signaling
- Insulin resistance development
- Decreased metabolic rate
- Sedation reducing physical activity

**Monitoring Requirements** demand systematic approaches to catch problems early. Baseline measurements include weight, waist circumference, blood pressure, fasting glucose, and lipid panel. The challenge lies in regular follow-up—many patients avoid blood draws or skip appointments when feeling well (97).

**Metabolic monitoring schedule** for antipsychotics:

- Baseline: weight, BMI, waist circumference, BP, glucose, lipids
- Month 1: weight, BP
- Month 2: weight
- Month 3: weight, BP, glucose, lipids
- Then quarterly for year 1, biannually thereafter
- Any significant weight gain: immediate metabolic reassessment

**Lab interpretation for non-prescribers** helps identify concerning changes:

- Weight gain >7% body weight warrants intervention
- Fasting glucose >100 mg/dL indicates prediabetes
- Triglycerides >150 mg/dL suggests metabolic syndrome
- Blood pressure >130/80 requires medical evaluation
- Waist circumference >40 inches (men) or >35 inches (women) indicates central obesity

**Intervention Strategies** should begin with prevention rather than reaction. **Lifestyle modifications that work** require practical, sustainable approaches:

Dietary interventions:

- Food diaries to identify eating patterns
- Smaller, frequent meals to manage increased appetite
- High-protein breakfasts reducing later cravings
- Avoiding simple carbohydrates that worsen insulin resistance
- Meal planning to prevent impulsive eating

Exercise programs:

- Starting with 10-minute walks, gradually increasing
- Finding enjoyable activities rather than "exercise"
- Using pedometers for objective feedback
- Group activities for accountability
- Addressing sedation that limits activity

**When to consider switching** depends on balancing psychiatric stability against medical risks. Generally, consider switching when:

- Weight gain exceeds 10% despite interventions
- Diabetes develops (though some continue with tight control)
- Lipids become severely abnormal
- Patient refuses medication due to weight gain
- Alternative medications with better metabolic profiles exist

**Clinical Pearl: The metformin option** offers hope for managing antipsychotic-induced weight gain. Metformin, traditionally used for diabetes, can prevent or reverse weight gain and metabolic abnormalities. Starting at 500 mg daily and increasing to 1000-2000 mg (divided doses) often helps. Benefits include:

- Average weight loss of 3-5 kg
- Improved insulin sensitivity
- Reduced appetite
- Lower cardiovascular risk
- Generally well-tolerated

Consider metformin early rather than waiting for severe metabolic dysfunction (98).

# Movement Disorders: Recognition and Response

Movement side effects from antipsychotics range from uncomfortable to disabling, sometimes persisting after medication discontinuation. Early recognition and appropriate management prevent long-term complications while maintaining psychiatric benefits.

**Acute EPS: The emergency presentations** include several distinct syndromes requiring different responses:

Acute dystonia presents dramatically with sustained muscle contractions causing abnormal postures. Patients might develop:

- Oculogyric crisis (eyes rolled back)
- Torticollis (twisted neck)
- Opisthotonus (arched back)
- Laryngeal dystonia (potentially fatal airway compromise)

Treatment requires immediate anticholinergic medication— benztropine 1-2 mg or diphenhydramine 25-50 mg IM/IV provides relief within minutes. Risk factors include young age, male gender, and high-potency antipsychotics (99).

Parkinsonism mimics Parkinson's disease with tremor, rigidity, and bradykinesia. Unlike acute dystonia, this develops over days to weeks. Management options:

- Dose reduction when possible
- Anticholinergics (though less effective than for dystonia)
- Switching to lower-EPS antipsychotics
- Adding amantadine for resistant cases

Akathisia causes subjective restlessness with objective fidgeting. Patients describe feeling like they need to crawl out of their skin. This distressing side effect increases suicide risk and medication non-adherence. Treatment:

- Beta-blockers (propranolol 10-40 mg TID)

- Benzodiazepines for acute relief
- Dose reduction or medication change
- Avoiding anticholinergics which rarely help

**Tardive Dyskinesia: Early recognition saves function** develops after months to years of antipsychotic exposure, potentially becoming irreversible. Classic signs include:

- Oro-buccal-lingual movements (tongue protrusion, lip smacking)
- Choreiform movements of limbs
- Truncal movements
- Respiratory dyskinesia (rare but serious)

Risk increases with:

- Longer treatment duration
- Higher cumulative doses
- Older age
- Female gender
- Mood disorders (higher risk than schizophrenia)
- First-generation antipsychotics

Prevention through using lowest effective doses and regular monitoring exceeds treatment effectiveness. Once identified, management includes:

- Switching to clozapine or quetiapine (lowest TD risk)
- VMAT2 inhibitors (valbenazine, deutetrabenazine) for established TD
- Avoiding anticholinergics which worsen TD
- Documenting carefully for medical-legal protection (100)

**AIMS Examination: Simplified for non-physicians** provides structured tardive dyskinesia assessment. The Abnormal Involuntary Movement Scale rates movements in different body regions from 0 (none) to 4 (severe). Key examination components:

1. Observe patient at rest in chair

2. Have patient protrude tongue twice
3. Check for tongue movements with mouth open
4. Tap thumb to fingers rapidly (activation maneuver)
5. Have patient stand and extend arms
6. Check gait
7. Observe during conversation

Any score of 2 (mild) in two areas or 3 (moderate) in one area warrants concern. Video recordings help document progression. Non-prescribers can perform basic AIMS screening, referring concerning findings for full evaluation (101).

## Case Study: Recognizing and Addressing Akathisia

Robert, a 52-year-old with bipolar disorder, started risperidone 2 mg for manic symptoms after refusing lithium due to past side effects. Within a week, his mania improved significantly, but he appeared increasingly agitated during therapy sessions.

"I can't sit still," he complained, constantly shifting position. "It's like having restless legs through my whole body. I pace all night—my wife says I'm wearing paths in the carpet." Observation revealed continuous leg movements, frequent position changes, and inability to remain seated for more than minutes.

The therapist recognized probable akathisia, distinct from manic restlessness by its physical discomfort and medication timing. Communication with the psychiatrist led to immediate intervention:

- Added propranolol 20 mg three times daily
- Reduced risperidone to 1.5 mg
- Provided clonazepam 0.5 mg for acute relief

Within days, Robert's restlessness decreased substantially. However, some akathisia persisted, leading to medication switch to quetiapine 400 mg, which controlled mania without movement side effects.

"That feeling was worse than the mania," Robert reflected. "I seriously considered stopping all medications. If you hadn't recognized what was happening, I would have quit treatment entirely."

## Practical Wisdom for Antipsychotic Use

Antipsychotics remain among psychiatry's most effective yet challenging medications. Their benefits extend far beyond treating psychosis, helping millions with bipolar disorder, depression, and severe anxiety. However, their risks demand respect and careful monitoring. Success requires balancing psychiatric improvement against medical consequences, always keeping patient preferences central.

The key lies in honest discussion about benefits and risks, careful selection based on individual factors, and vigilant monitoring for both therapeutic response and adverse effects. When used thoughtfully, antipsychotics transform lives. When used carelessly, they cause significant harm. Understanding their complexities empowers clinicians to maximize benefits while minimizing risks.

### Key Takeaways

- Antipsychotics treat numerous conditions beyond schizophrenia including bipolar disorder, treatment-resistant depression, and severe anxiety
- First-generation antipsychotics primarily block dopamine while second-generation agents affect multiple neurotransmitter systems
- Metabolic side effects follow a hierarchy with olanzapine and clozapine causing most weight gain
- Regular monitoring of weight, glucose, and lipids catches metabolic problems early
- Metformin can prevent or reverse antipsychotic-induced weight gain and metabolic dysfunction

- Movement disorders range from acute dystonia requiring emergency treatment to tardive dyskinesia potentially becoming permanent
- Akathisia causes severe subjective distress often leading to medication discontinuation
- AIMS examinations should be performed regularly to detect early tardive dyskinesia
- Individual medication selection depends on symptom profile, side effect history, and patient preferences
- Success requires ongoing risk-benefit assessment and open communication about side effects

# Chapter 7: Anxiety Medications - Calming the Storm

Anxiety disorders affect 40 million adults annually, making them the most common mental health conditions. Yet medication treatment for anxiety remains controversial, balancing rapid relief against dependence risks. Understanding the full spectrum of anti-anxiety medications—from benzodiazepines to novel alternatives—helps clinicians provide effective treatment while minimizing harm.

## Benzodiazepines: Benefits and Risks

For over 60 years, benzodiazepines have provided rapid anxiety relief when other treatments fail or work too slowly. Their effectiveness is undeniable, yet their risks demand careful consideration and monitoring. Understanding both aspects helps clinicians use these medications appropriately.

**How They Work: GABA enhancement explained** through a simple lock-and-key analogy. GABA, the brain's main inhibitory neurotransmitter, acts like a master brake pedal slowing overactive circuits. Benzodiazepines don't create more GABA—instead, they make existing GABA work better. Think of GABA as a key that opens chloride channels (doors) in neurons. Benzodiazepines oil these locks, making the doors open more easily and stay open longer. This enhanced inhibition calms anxiety within 30-60 minutes (102).

Different benzodiazepines bind to slightly different sites on GABA receptors, explaining their varied effects:

- Alpha-1 subunits: sedation and amnesia
- Alpha-2 and 3 subunits: anxiety reduction and muscle relaxation
- Alpha-5 subunits: cognitive effects

This knowledge drives development of selective medications targeting anxiety without sedation, though none have yet matched benzodiazepines' effectiveness.

**Short vs. Long-Acting: Choosing wisely** requires matching medication pharmacokinetics to clinical needs:

Short-acting benzodiazepines:

- Alprazolam (Xanax): 6-12 hour duration
- Lorazepam (Ativan): 10-20 hour duration
- Oxazepam (Serax): 4-15 hour duration

Long-acting benzodiazepines:

- Clonazepam (Klonopin): 18-50 hour duration
- Diazepam (Valium): 20-100 hour duration
- Chlordiazepoxide (Librium): 5-30 hour duration

Short-acting medications provide rapid relief for panic attacks or procedural anxiety but require multiple daily doses and cause more rebound anxiety. Long-acting options offer smoother coverage with less frequent dosing but accumulate in elderly patients or those with liver disease (103).

**Addiction and Dependence** represent benzodiazepines' greatest challenge, often misunderstood by both clinicians and patients. Physical dependence—neuroadaptation requiring continued use to prevent withdrawal—occurs in virtually all regular users within weeks. This differs from addiction, which involves compulsive use despite harm, affecting only 5-10% of prescribed users (104).

**Risk factors identification** helps predict who might develop problematic use:

- Personal or family history of substance use disorders
- History of seeking early refills or dose escalation
- Concurrent use of alcohol or other substances
- Personality disorders, particularly cluster B

- High-dose or short-acting benzodiazepine use
- Obtaining prescriptions from multiple providers

**Safe prescribing practices** minimize risks while providing needed relief:

1. Clear treatment agreements specifying duration and goals
2. Regular reassessment of continued need
3. Avoiding concurrent opioids when possible
4. Using lowest effective doses
5. Preferring longer-acting agents for chronic anxiety
6. Monitoring for aberrant behaviors
7. Documenting risk-benefit discussions

**Clinical Pearl: The 2-4 week rule** provides practical guidance for preventing dependence. For acute anxiety or adjustment disorders, limit benzodiazepines to 2-4 weeks while establishing longer-term treatments. This timeframe provides relief while minimizing dependence risk. Exceptions exist—panic disorder might require longer treatment— but time-limited use should be the default (105).

**Tapering Strategies** prevent withdrawal symptoms that can be severe and prolonged. Abrupt discontinuation after regular use causes:

- Rebound anxiety exceeding original symptoms
- Insomnia, often severe
- Tremor and muscle tension
- Perceptual disturbances
- Seizures in severe cases

**The Ashton Manual simplified** provides evidence-based tapering guidance. Key principles include:

- Slow tapering over weeks to months
- 10% dose reductions every 1-2 weeks
- Switching short-acting to long-acting benzodiazepines first
- Patient-controlled tapering pace
- Adjunctive medications for withdrawal symptoms
- Psychological support throughout

For example, tapering alprazolam 2 mg daily:

1. Convert to diazepam equivalent (20 mg)
2. Reduce by 2 mg every 2 weeks initially
3. Slow to 1 mg reductions below 10 mg
4. May take 3-6 months total

**Benzodiazepine equivalency table** guides conversions:

- Alprazolam 0.5 mg = Diazepam 5 mg
- Lorazepam 1 mg = Diazepam 10 mg
- Clonazepam 0.5 mg = Diazepam 10 mg
- Temazepam 20 mg = Diazepam 10 mg

These equivalencies approximate—individual responses vary significantly (106).

## Case Vignette: Helping James Taper Off Xanax

James, a 41-year-old sales manager, started alprazolam during his divorce three years ago. "My doctor said it would help temporarily," he explained. Initially taking 0.5 mg as needed, he now required 2 mg three times daily to prevent "horrible anxiety."

Attempted self-tapering triggered severe symptoms: "I cut my dose in half and thought I was dying—heart racing, sweating, couldn't think straight. The anxiety was ten times worse than before I started." His physician referred him for structured tapering.

Assessment revealed:

- Physical dependence without addiction behaviors
- Motivated for discontinuation
- Stable psychosocial situation
- No concurrent substance use
- Previous anxiety well-controlled without medication

The tapering plan:

1. Education about withdrawal expectations
2. Switch to diazepam 60 mg daily (equivalent dose)
3. Weekly 5 mg reductions to 40 mg
4. Biweekly 5 mg reductions to 20 mg
5. Weekly 2 mg reductions to 10 mg
6. Weekly 1 mg reductions to cessation
7. CBT for anxiety management throughout

James experienced manageable symptoms—mild anxiety, insomnia, muscle tension—but never severe withdrawal. The entire taper took 5 months. Six months post-discontinuation, he remained benzodiazepine-free using learned coping strategies.

"I wish I'd never started," James reflected, "but I'm proud I got off them safely. The slow taper made all the difference—my previous attempts were way too fast."

## Alternative Anxiolytics

Growing awareness of benzodiazepine risks drives interest in alternative anxiety medications. While generally less rapidly effective, these options provide sustainable anxiety relief without dependence risk.

**Buspirone: The slow and steady option** works through serotonin 5-HT1A partial agonism—completely different from benzodiazepines. Think of it as gradually resetting the anxiety thermostat rather than acutely suppressing symptoms. Starting at 5 mg twice daily and increasing to 15-30 mg twice daily, buspirone requires 2-4 weeks for full effect (107).

Advantages include:

- No dependence or withdrawal
- No sedation or cognitive impairment
- No interaction with alcohol
- May improve depression symptoms
- Safe in elderly patients

Disadvantages:

- Delayed onset frustrates anxious patients
- Less effective for severe anxiety
- No benefit for acute panic
- Requires consistent daily dosing
- Dizziness and nausea common initially

Patient selection matters—buspirone works best for generalized anxiety without panic attacks in benzodiazepine-naive patients. Those expecting immediate relief like benzodiazepines inevitably feel disappointed.

**Hydroxyzine: Fast-acting without addiction** provides rapid anxiety relief through antihistamine properties. Available doses of 25-100 mg work within 30-60 minutes, lasting 4-6 hours. Unlike benzodiazepines, hydroxyzine causes no dependence regardless of use duration (108).

Clinical uses include:

- Acute anxiety episodes
- Preoperative anxiety
- Insomnia secondary to anxiety
- Augmentation of other anxiolytics
- Bridge therapy while starting SSRIs

Side effects center on antihistamine properties: sedation, dry mouth, constipation, blurred vision. Elderly patients show particular sensitivity. Despite limitations, hydroxyzine offers valuable acute relief without addiction risk.

**Beta-blockers: For performance anxiety** target physical anxiety symptoms rather than psychological distress. Propranolol 10-40 mg taken 30-60 minutes before anxiety-provoking situations reduces:

- Rapid heartbeat
- Tremor
- Sweating

- Blushing
- Voice quavering

Musicians, public speakers, and test-takers particularly benefit. Beta-blockers don't reduce cognitive anxiety—racing thoughts persist—but eliminating physical symptoms often breaks the anxiety spiral. Contraindications include asthma, bradycardia, and certain heart conditions (109).

**Off-label Options: Gabapentin and pregabalin** originally developed for epilepsy, show increasing evidence for anxiety disorders. Gabapentin doses of 300-1800 mg daily (divided TID) help generalized anxiety, while pregabalin 150-600 mg daily (divided BID) has European approval for anxiety.

Mechanisms involve:

- Reducing glutamate release
- Enhancing GABA synthesis
- Modulating calcium channels
- Decreasing neuronal excitability

Benefits include rapid onset (days), no metabolic effects, and usefulness for comorbid pain. Concerns include sedation, weight gain, and emerging evidence of abuse potential in some populations (110).

## Case Study: Choosing Non-Addictive Anxiety Treatment

Lisa, a 35-year-old teacher, developed severe anxiety after witnessing school violence. "I can't stop thinking about it," she reported. "My heart races constantly, I'm too anxious to teach, and I haven't slept well in months." Her primary care physician offered benzodiazepines, but Lisa's father struggled with alcohol—she feared addiction.

Comprehensive assessment revealed:

- Generalized anxiety with panic attacks
- Hypervigilance and re-experiencing symptoms

67

- Significant insomnia
- No substance use history
- Strong family support
- Motivated for therapy

The treatment plan combined medication and therapy:

1. Started hydroxyzine 50 mg for acute anxiety and sleep
2. Initiated sertraline 25 mg, titrating slowly
3. Added propranolol 20 mg before teaching
4. Weekly CBT focusing on trauma processing

Hydroxyzine provided immediate relief without dependence risk. "Finally, I could breathe again," Lisa noted. Sertraline reached 100 mg over 6 weeks with good anxiety reduction. Propranolol eliminated physical symptoms during teaching, restoring confidence.

Three months later, Lisa tapered hydroxyzine successfully, maintaining improvement with sertraline and therapy. One year post-trauma, she remained stable without benzodiazepines.

"I'm grateful we found alternatives," she reflected. "With my family history, benzodiazepines would have been risky. The combination approach took longer but feels sustainable."

## Building Comprehensive Treatment

Anxiety medication works best within comprehensive treatment including therapy, lifestyle modifications, and social support. Medications provide a window of reduced symptoms, allowing patients to engage in therapy and build lasting coping skills. The goal isn't indefinite medication but rather achieving remission that persists after tapering.

Understanding each medication's unique properties, appropriate uses, and limitations empowers informed treatment decisions. While benzodiazepines remain valuable for specific situations, alternative anxiolytics offer sustainable relief without dependence risks. Success requires matching medication choice to individual patient factors while always considering long-term outcomes over short-term relief.

**Key Takeaways**

- Benzodiazepines enhance GABA function providing rapid anxiety relief within 30-60 minutes
- Physical dependence develops in weeks with regular use, distinct from addiction
- Safe prescribing involves time-limited use, clear agreements, and regular reassessment
- Tapering must proceed slowly over months to prevent severe withdrawal
- Buspirone offers non-addictive anxiety treatment but requires 2-4 weeks for effect
- Hydroxyzine provides rapid relief without dependence risk though causes sedation
- Beta-blockers effectively treat performance anxiety by reducing physical symptoms
- Gabapentin and pregabalin show promise for anxiety with rapid onset and no metabolic effects
- Alternative anxiolytics generally work best for mild-moderate anxiety without panic attacks
- Comprehensive treatment combining medication with therapy optimizes long-term outcomes

# Chapter 8: Specialty Medications

Beyond the major medication classes, several specialized categories address specific conditions like ADHD, insomnia, and cognitive decline. These medications often require particular expertise in dosing, monitoring, and managing unique side effects. Understanding their proper use helps clinicians support patients with these challenging conditions while avoiding common pitfalls.

## ADHD Medications

Attention-deficit/hyperactivity disorder affects 5% of children and 2.5% of adults, causing significant functional impairment across life domains. Medication treatment can dramatically improve outcomes, but stimulants' controlled substance status and abuse potential create clinical complexities requiring careful management.

**Stimulants: Turning up the focus dial** work by increasing dopamine and norepinephrine in prefrontal circuits responsible for attention and executive function. Think of ADHD as having a radio with poor reception—stimulants boost the signal strength, bringing clarity to mental static. Effects begin within 30-60 minutes, providing immediate improvement unlike most psychiatric medications (111).

**Methylphenidate vs. amphetamines** represent two stimulant families with subtle but important differences:

Methylphenidate-based medications:

- Ritalin, Concerta, Focalin, Daytrana patch
- Block dopamine and norepinephrine reuptake
- Duration varies: 3-4 hours (immediate-release) to 12 hours (Concerta)
- Generally fewer mood effects
- Lower abuse potential than amphetamines

Amphetamine-based medications:

- Adderall, Vyvanse, Dexedrine
- Block reuptake AND increase neurotransmitter release
- More potent mg-per-mg than methylphenidate
- Higher risk of mood changes and anxiety
- Vyvanse's prodrug design reduces abuse potential

Individual responses vary significantly—some patients respond only to one family. Trial and error often necessary to find optimal medication (112).

**Abuse potential and monitoring** requires balancing access for legitimate patients against diversion risks. Warning signs include:

- Requests for early refills
- "Lost" prescriptions
- Specific medication demands
- Dose escalation without consultation
- Obtaining stimulants from multiple providers

Monitoring strategies:

- Prescription drug monitoring program checks
- Random drug screens (ensuring prescribed medication present)
- Pill counts for concerning patients
- Clear treatment agreements
- Regular assessment of continued need
- Documentation of functional improvement

Most ADHD patients use stimulants appropriately, but vigilance prevents problems (113).

**Dosing and titration guide** follows "start low, go slow" principles:

Methylphenidate immediate-release:

- Start: 5 mg twice daily
- Increase: 5-10 mg weekly
- Maximum: 60 mg daily divided

Methylphenidate extended-release (Concerta):

- Start: 18 mg morning
- Increase: 18 mg weekly
- Maximum: 72 mg daily

Amphetamine mixed salts immediate-release:

- Start: 5 mg once or twice daily
- Increase: 5 mg weekly
- Maximum: 40 mg daily

Amphetamine mixed salts extended-release:

- Start: 10-20 mg morning
- Increase: 10 mg weekly
- Maximum: 30 mg daily (adults)

Titrate based on symptom control and side effects, not mg/kg calculations (114).

## Case Example 1: The Struggling Student

Mark, a 19-year-old college sophomore, sought evaluation after nearly failing freshman year. "I study for hours but can't focus," he explained. "I read the same page over and over. In lectures, my mind wanders constantly." Testing confirmed ADHD, predominantly inattentive type.

Starting methylphenidate 5 mg twice daily produced dramatic improvement: "It's like someone cleaned my mental windshield." Titration to 10 mg three times daily optimized focus without side effects. Grades improved from D's to B's within one semester.

However, Mark soon requested Adderall, claiming methylphenidate "stopped working." Investigation revealed he'd been sharing medication with roommates and taking extra doses before exams. This misuse pattern required intervention:

- Switching to Concerta (harder to abuse due to OROS delivery system)
- Weekly dispensing initially
- Concurrent therapy addressing underlying anxiety
- Clear boundaries about medication sharing

With structure and support, Mark stabilized on appropriate treatment without further misuse.

**Non-stimulants: When stimulants aren't appropriate** provide alternatives for patients with substance abuse history, cardiovascular concerns, or stimulant intolerance. While less immediately effective than stimulants, they offer sustainable improvement without abuse potential (115).

Atomoxetine (Strattera):

- Selective norepinephrine reuptake inhibitor
- Start 40 mg daily, increase to 80-100 mg
- Takes 4-6 weeks for full effect
- No abuse potential or controlled status
- Side effects: nausea, decreased appetite, sexual dysfunction

Guanfacine (Intuniv) and clonidine (Kapvay):

- Alpha-2 agonists reducing norepinephrine release
- Particularly helpful for hyperactivity/impulsivity
- Sedation common initially
- Monitor blood pressure and heart rate
- Often combined with stimulants

Bupropion off-label:

- Mild benefit for ADHD symptoms
- Helpful when depression coexists
- Activating properties aid concentration
- Lower efficacy than approved ADHD medications

**Clinical Pearl: Managing appetite suppression** addresses stimulants' most common side effect. Strategies include:

- Eating substantial breakfast before medication
- Scheduling "medication holidays" on weekends
- Liquid nutrition supplements for weight loss
- Dose timing to allow dinner appetite
- Switching preparations (some suppress appetite less)
- Adding cyproheptadine for severe cases

Most patients adapt within weeks, but monitoring weight remains essential, especially in children (116).

## Sleep Medications

Insomnia affects one-third of adults, with 10% experiencing chronic sleep difficulties significantly impairing daytime function. While cognitive-behavioral therapy for insomnia (CBT-I) provides first-line treatment, medications offer short-term relief during acute stress or while establishing behavioral changes.

**Z-drugs: Not quite benzodiazepines** include zolpidem (Ambien), eszopiclone (Lunesta), and zaleplon (Sonata). Despite different chemical structures than benzodiazepines, they work through similar GABA mechanisms but with greater selectivity for sleep-promoting receptors. This selectivity theoretically reduces dependence risk and daytime sedation, though real-world experience suggests similar concerns (117).

Zolpidem characteristics:

- Rapid onset (15-30 minutes)
- Short duration (6-8 hours)
- Doses: 5-10 mg (5 mg in women, elderly)
- Less muscle relaxation than benzodiazepines
- Unusual side effects: sleep eating, sleep driving

Eszopiclone features:

- Longer half-life permitting middle-night dosing
- FDA approved for long-term use
- Metallic taste common
- Doses: 1-3 mg

Zaleplon properties:

- Ultra-short acting (4 hours)
- Useful for sleep initiation only
- Can be taken middle-of-night if 4+ hours remain
- Doses: 5-10 mg

**Melatonin and alternatives** offer gentler approaches to sleep difficulties:

Melatonin:

- Hormone regulating circadian rhythms
- Most effective for jet lag, shift work
- Doses: 0.5-5 mg (lower often more effective)
- Take 2-3 hours before desired bedtime
- Minimal side effects or dependence

Ramelteon (Rozerem):

- Melatonin receptor agonist
- No abuse potential
- Modest efficacy for sleep initiation
- Safe in elderly and substance abuse history

Trazodone off-label:

- Sedating antidepressant
- Doses: 25-100 mg for sleep
- No tolerance or dependence
- Side effects: morning grogginess, priapism (rare)

Doxepin (Silenor):

- Tricyclic antidepressant at sub-antidepressant doses
- 3-6 mg for sleep maintenance
- Particularly helpful for early morning awakening

**Complex sleep behaviors: The FDA warnings explained** highlight serious risks with sedative-hypnotics. Patients report activities with no memory:

- Sleep driving
- Preparing and eating food
- Making phone calls
- Sexual activity

Risk factors include:

- Higher doses
- Concurrent alcohol or CNS depressants
- Taking medication without immediately going to bed
- Previous parasomnia history

FDA requires boxed warnings and contraindications for patients with previous complex sleep behaviors. Education about never taking sleep medications unless able to get full night's sleep proves critical (118).

## Case Vignette: Addressing Chronic Insomnia Safely

Patricia, a 58-year-old executive, requested "something strong for sleep" after months of insomnia following her husband's death. "I've tried everything—melatonin, Benadryl, three glasses of wine. Nothing works. I need real sleep medication."

Assessment revealed:

- Sleep initiation and maintenance problems
- Grief with mild depression
- No substance abuse history
- Previous good response to therapy
- Motivated for non-medication approaches

Treatment approach:

1. Education about sleep hygiene and grief's impact
2. Referral for grief counseling
3. Short-term zolpidem 5 mg with clear limits
4. Concurrent CBT-I referral
5. Plan for medication taper after 4 weeks

Patricia initially resisted CBT-I: "I don't have time for all those sleep rules." However, combining immediate relief from zolpidem with gradual behavioral changes proved effective. After four weeks, she tapered zolpidem while maintaining improved sleep through CBT-I techniques.

Six months later: "I sleep better now than before my husband died. Those behavioral changes seemed silly but really work. I'm glad we didn't just continue the sleeping pills indefinitely."

## Cognitive Enhancers

As populations age globally, demand increases for medications to prevent or treat cognitive decline. While several drugs show modest benefits for dementia, unrealistic expectations often lead to disappointment. Understanding what these medications can and cannot do helps set appropriate goals.

**For dementia: Realistic expectations** require honest discussion about limited benefits. Current medications don't cure or stop Alzheimer's disease—they temporarily improve symptoms or slow decline by months, not years. Families hoping for dramatic improvement inevitably feel disappointed without proper education (119).

Cholinesterase inhibitors:

- Donepezil (Aricept): 5-10 mg daily
- Rivastigmine (Exelon): patch or capsules
- Galantamine (Razadyne): 8-24 mg daily

These medications boost acetylcholine by preventing breakdown, modestly improving memory and function in mild-moderate dementia. Side effects include nausea, diarrhea, and bradycardia.

Memantine (Namenda):

- NMDA receptor antagonist
- For moderate-severe dementia
- 5-20 mg daily (titrated slowly)
- Often combined with cholinesterase inhibitors
- Better tolerated than cholinesterase inhibitors

**Mechanisms and modest benefits** help families understand reasonable expectations:

- 2-3 point improvement on 70-point cognitive scales
- 6-12 month delay in nursing home placement
- Temporary stabilization of function
- Individual responses vary dramatically
- Not everyone benefits measurably

Benefits appear most pronounced in:

- Early-stage disease
- Consistent medication adherence
- Absence of other medical complications
- Strong family support systems

**When to start, when to stop** creates difficult decisions for families and clinicians:

Starting considerations:

- Mild-moderate Alzheimer's disease confirmed
- Realistic expectations established
- Ability to monitor for side effects
- Family understanding of modest benefits
- Cost-benefit discussion completed

Stopping considerations:

- Advanced dementia (unable to recognize family)
- Significant side effects outweighing benefits
- No apparent benefit after adequate trial
- Swallowing difficulties developing
- Quality of life focus in terminal stages

The decision to stop often proves harder than starting, requiring sensitive family discussions about shifting goals from treatment to comfort (120).

## Case Example 2: Managing Expectations

George, a 72-year-old retired engineer, received an Alzheimer's diagnosis after two years of memory complaints. His daughter arrived with printed research: "I want him on everything—Aricept, Namenda, plus those new antibody drugs. We're going to beat this."

Careful education addressed unrealistic expectations:

- Current medications provide modest, temporary benefits
- No available treatment stops or reverses Alzheimer's
- Side effects might outweigh benefits
- Newer treatments show limited real-world effectiveness

Starting donepezil 5 mg caused significant nausea initially but improved with food. After titrating to 10 mg, George showed mild improvement—remembering grandchildren's names, less repetitive questions. His daughter initially felt disappointed: "I thought he'd be back to normal."

Reframing success helped: "He's maintaining function longer than without treatment. Every good day matters." The family focused on quality time while medication provided modest support.

Two years later, with advancing disease, the family decided to discontinue donepezil: "It served its purpose, giving us more good months. Now comfort matters most."

## Practical Perspectives on Specialty Medications

Specialty psychiatric medications serve important roles for specific conditions, but their use requires particular knowledge and careful monitoring. Stimulants transform ADHD treatment but demand vigilance against misuse. Sleep medications provide short-term relief while behavioral interventions take effect. Cognitive enhancers offer modest benefits for dementia when expectations remain realistic.

Success with these medications requires:

- Clear treatment goals and realistic expectations
- Regular monitoring for efficacy and side effects
- Integration with non-medication interventions
- Flexibility to adjust or discontinue based on response
- Honest communication about benefits and limitations

Understanding each medication's appropriate role prevents both overuse and underutilization, helping patients achieve optimal outcomes while minimizing risks.

### Key Takeaways

- Stimulants rapidly improve ADHD symptoms by enhancing dopamine and norepinephrine signaling
- Methylphenidate and amphetamines show similar efficacy but individual responses vary
- Non-stimulant ADHD medications provide alternatives for those with substance abuse history or stimulant intolerance
- Z-drugs work similarly to benzodiazepines for sleep but carry risks of complex sleep behaviors
- Melatonin and behavioral interventions offer safer long-term insomnia management

- Cognitive enhancers provide modest, temporary benefits for dementia, not cure or reversal
- Realistic expectations prevent disappointment with specialty medications' limited effects
- Monitoring requirements vary by medication class but remain essential for safety
- Integration with behavioral interventions optimizes outcomes across all specialty medication categories
- Individual response variability necessitates flexible, patient-centered approaches

# Chapter 9: Drug Interactions and Safety

Drug interactions kill more people annually than car accidents, yet most are preventable with basic knowledge and systematic checking. Every psychiatric medication travels through the body's metabolic highways, competing for space with other drugs, foods, and supplements. Understanding these interactions transforms abstract warnings into practical safety measures that protect patients from dangerous combinations while maximizing therapeutic benefits.

## CYP450 System Simplified

The cytochrome P450 system sounds intimidating, but think of it as your liver's highway system with multiple lanes processing different medications. Just as rush-hour traffic creates delays when too many cars use the same route, medications can create "traffic jams" in these metabolic pathways, causing dangerous accumulations or treatment failures.

**The "highway system" of drug metabolism** consists of several major routes, each named with numbers and letters like CYP3A4, CYP2D6, and CYP2C19. These enzymes work like toll booths processing medications—some work faster, others slower, and certain drugs can shut down entire lanes or speed up traffic flow.

CYP3A4 represents the busiest highway, processing over 50% of all medications. Common psychiatric drugs using this route include:

- Alprazolam, midazolam, triazolam (benzodiazepines)
- Quetiapine, lurasidone, aripiprazole (antipsychotics)
- Buspirone (anxiolytic)
- Carbamazepine (mood stabilizer)

CYP2D6 acts as a specialized route for many psychiatric medications:

- Most SSRIs (especially fluoxetine and paroxetine)
- Tricyclic antidepressants
- Venlafaxine, duloxetine (SNRIs)

- Risperidone, aripiprazole (antipsychotics)
- Atomoxetine (ADHD medication)

CYP2C19 handles a smaller but important group:

- Citalopram, escitalopram (SSRIs)
- Diazepam (benzodiazepine)
- Some tricyclic antidepressants

Understanding which medications use which pathways predicts interactions. When two drugs compete for the same enzyme, one inevitably gets processed more slowly, potentially reaching toxic levels (121).

**Major interactions to memorize** include combinations that frequently cause problems in clinical practice:

**Fluoxetine + anything metabolized by CYP2D6** creates significant issues. Fluoxetine powerfully inhibits CYP2D6 for weeks after discontinuation due to its long half-life. Adding risperidone to fluoxetine can triple risperidone levels, causing severe side effects. Similarly, fluoxetine can double tricyclic antidepressant levels, risking cardiac toxicity.

**Carbamazepine + oral contraceptives** represents a critical interaction often missed. Carbamazepine powerfully induces CYP3A4, speeding up contraceptive metabolism and causing breakthrough pregnancies. Women taking carbamazepine need alternative birth control methods or significantly higher contraceptive doses.

**Multiple serotonergic medications** create additive effects rather than true metabolic interactions. Combining SSRIs with tramadol, triptans, linezolid, or St. John's Wort risks serotonin syndrome through different mechanisms all increasing serotonin activity.

**Smoking + clozapine or olanzapine** demonstrates environmental interactions. Cigarette smoke induces CYP1A2, requiring 50% higher doses in smokers. Hospitalized patients forced to quit smoking can develop toxicity if doses aren't reduced promptly (122).

**Common CYP interactions** follow predictable patterns:

Strong CYP3A4 inhibitors (increasing other drug levels):

- Ketoconazole, itraconazole (antifungals)
- Clarithromycin, erythromycin (antibiotics)
- Grapefruit juice (even small amounts)
- HIV protease inhibitors

Strong CYP3A4 inducers (decreasing other drug levels):

- Carbamazepine, phenytoin (anticonvulsants)
- Rifampin (antibiotic)
- St. John's Wort (supplement)
- Modafinil (wakefulness agent)

Strong CYP2D6 inhibitors:

- Fluoxetine, paroxetine (SSRIs)
- Bupropion (antidepressant)
- Quinidine (antiarrhythmic)

The key to managing interactions lies not in memorizing every combination but understanding principles and checking interactions systematically with each medication change.

## Case Example 1: The Dangerous Combination

Margaret, a 58-year-old teacher, took venlafaxine 150 mg for depression with excellent response. She developed a urinary tract infection and received ciprofloxacin from urgent care. Within two days, she experienced severe nausea, tremor, and confusion. Her husband found her disoriented with dilated pupils and profuse sweating.

The emergency department diagnosed serotonin syndrome from venlafaxine-ciprofloxacin interaction. While not commonly recognized, ciprofloxacin inhibits CYP1A2 and CYP3A4, increasing venlafaxine levels. Combined with venlafaxine's serotonergic effects, this triggered moderate serotonin syndrome.

Treatment included:

- Discontinuing both medications
- Supportive care with IV fluids
- Benzodiazepines for agitation
- Cyproheptadine for serotonin antagonism

Margaret recovered fully within 48 hours but required antibiotic adjustment and temporary venlafaxine dose reduction. This case illustrates how common medications can interact dangerously when prescribers work in isolation.

## Serotonin Syndrome Deep Dive

Serotonin syndrome progresses from mild discomfort to life-threatening emergency rapidly, making early recognition critical. Unlike many drug reactions developing over days or weeks, serotonin syndrome can escalate within hours, particularly after medication changes or overdoses.

**Recognition in non-medical settings** requires awareness of the classic triad: mental status changes, autonomic hyperactivity, and neuromuscular abnormalities. Think of it as serotonin "overdose" affecting the entire nervous system simultaneously.

Mental status changes often appear first:

- Anxiety, agitation, restlessness
- Confusion, disorientation
- Hypomania or delirium
- Hallucinations in severe cases

Autonomic hyperactivity creates physical symptoms:

- Hyperthermia (fever)
- Diaphoresis (profuse sweating)
- Tachycardia (rapid heart rate)
- Hypertension or labile blood pressure
- Mydriasis (dilated pupils)
- Flushing

Neuromuscular abnormalities distinguish serotonin syndrome from other conditions:

- Tremor
- Myoclonus (muscle jerks)
- Hyperreflexia (overactive reflexes)
- Muscle rigidity
- Bilateral Babinski signs
- Ocular clonus (rhythmic eye movements)

The Hunter Serotonin Toxicity Criteria provides diagnostic accuracy. Presence of a serotonergic agent plus ONE of the following confirms diagnosis:

- Spontaneous clonus
- Inducible clonus plus agitation or diaphoresis
- Ocular clonus plus agitation or diaphoresis
- Tremor plus hyperreflexia
- Hypertonia plus temperature >38°C plus clonus (123).

**What to do while waiting for EMS** can significantly impact outcomes:

1. **Stop all serotonergic medications immediately** - every minute counts
2. **Cool the patient** - remove excess clothing, apply cool (not cold) compresses
3. **Maintain hydration** - offer water if patient can swallow safely

4. **Monitor vital signs** if possible - temperature, pulse, blood pressure
5. **Keep patient calm** - agitation worsens symptoms
6. **Document medications** - create list of all medications, doses, and timing
7. **Prevent injury** - muscle jerks can cause falls or trauma

Never give additional medications unless directed by emergency services. Avoid physical restraints which can worsen hyperthermia. If patient takes benzodiazepines regularly, these can be continued as they may help (124).

## Case Example 2: The Supplement Surprise

David, a 42-year-old engineer, took sertraline 100 mg for depression. Frustrated with persistent fatigue, he started multiple "natural" supplements from a health food store: St. John's Wort, SAM-e, 5-HTP, and L-tryptophan. "They're natural, so they must be safe," he reasoned.

Within three days, his wife noticed concerning changes during a therapy session. David appeared flushed, tremulous, and spoke rapidly with obvious confusion. When he stood, he nearly fell due to leg jerking. Temperature measured 101.2°F.

Recognition of probable serotonin syndrome prompted immediate action:

- Called 911 with clear description of symptoms
- Gathered all medications and supplements
- Kept David seated and calm
- Applied cool cloths to forehead and neck
- Documented symptom timeline

The emergency department confirmed moderate serotonin syndrome. All supplements contained serotonergic compounds that combined dangerously with sertraline. Treatment included cyproheptadine and supportive care with full recovery in 36 hours.

This case highlights how "natural" doesn't mean safe, especially when combined with prescription serotonergic medications.

## QT Prolongation: The Heart Rhythm Risk

QT prolongation represents a silent danger with psychiatric medications—invisible without EKG monitoring yet potentially fatal. The QT interval measures the heart's electrical recharge time. When prolonged, it creates risk for torsades de pointes, a chaotic rhythm causing sudden death.

Multiple psychiatric medications prolong QT interval to varying degrees:

- High risk: thioridazine, ziprasidone, IV haloperidol
- Moderate risk: citalopram (dose-dependent), chlorpromazine
- Lower risk: most other antipsychotics and antidepressants

Risk factors multiply danger:

- Female sex (longer baseline QT)
- Age over 65
- Electrolyte abnormalities (low potassium, magnesium)
- Heart disease
- Congenital long QT syndrome
- Multiple QT-prolonging drugs
- Liver or kidney disease

Citalopram requires special attention after FDA warnings. Maximum doses are:

- 40 mg daily for most adults
- 20 mg daily for patients over 60
- 20 mg daily with CYP2C19 inhibitors

Monitoring recommendations:

- Baseline EKG for high-risk medications or patients

- Electrolyte checks with diuretics or eating disorders
- Follow-up EKG with dose increases
- Immediate EKG for syncope or palpitations

QTc (corrected QT) interpretation:

- Normal: <440 ms (men), <460 ms (women)
- Borderline: 440-500 ms
- High risk: >500 ms or increase >60 ms from baseline (125).

## Clinical Scenarios: Interaction Management in Practice

Real-world interaction management requires systematic approaches adapted to common clinical situations. These scenarios illustrate practical applications of interaction knowledge.

**Scenario 1: The Anxious Cardiac Patient** Robert, 67, has coronary artery disease, atrial fibrillation, and new-onset anxiety. He takes:

- Metoprolol for blood pressure
- Amiodarone for atrial fibrillation
- Warfarin for stroke prevention
- Simvastatin for cholesterol

His cardiologist refers for anxiety management, suggesting "something mild."

Interaction analysis reveals:

- Amiodarone inhibits multiple CYP enzymes and prolongs QT
- Warfarin interacts with numerous psychiatric medications
- Elderly status increases sensitivity

Safe approach:

- Avoid citalopram (QT prolongation with amiodarone)
- Avoid benzodiazepines (fall risk with warfarin)
- Choose sertraline 25 mg (minimal CYP interactions)

- Monitor INR closely initially
- Consider buspirone if SSRI ineffective

**Scenario 2: The Polysubstance User** Jessica, 28, enters treatment for opioid and benzodiazepine dependence. She takes:

- Methadone 80 mg daily
- Clonazepam 2 mg twice daily (tapering)
- Birth control pills
- Gabapentin for anxiety

She reports severe depression needing treatment.

Interaction concerns:

- Methadone prolongs QT and uses CYP3A4
- Benzodiazepine taper complicates sedating medications
- Need to maintain birth control efficacy

Safe management:

- Obtain baseline EKG (methadone QT risk)
- Avoid additional QT prolongers
- Choose bupropion (no sedation, helps addiction)
- Continue gabapentin for anxiety
- Monitor closely during benzodiazepine taper

**Scenario 3: The Complex Medical Patient** William, 72, has diabetes, chronic pain, and depression. Medications include:

- Gabapentin 300 mg three times daily
- Tramadol 50 mg four times daily
- Metformin 1000 mg twice daily
- Lisinopril 20 mg daily
- Duloxetine just prescribed for depression/pain

Interaction analysis:

- Tramadol + duloxetine = high serotonin syndrome risk
- Both medications help pain
- Elderly with multiple conditions

Resolution:

- Discontinue tramadol before starting duloxetine
- Use acetaminophen for breakthrough pain
- Start duloxetine 30 mg daily
- Monitor for serotonin symptoms
- Consider adding pregabalin if pain control inadequate

These scenarios demonstrate how systematic interaction assessment prevents adverse events while achieving therapeutic goals.

## Case Example 3: The Hidden Interaction

Linda, 45, stable on lithium for bipolar disorder, developed severe headaches. Her neurologist prescribed sumatriptan for migraines and added propranolol for prevention. Within a week, Linda felt "off"— tremulous, nauseated, with worsening concentration.

Neither specialist considered interactions with lithium. Investigation revealed:

- Propranolol masked lithium toxicity symptoms (tremor, tachycardia)
- Sumatriptan theoretical risk of serotonin syndrome with lithium
- Dehydration from repeated vomiting concentrated lithium

Lithium level returned at 1.4 mEq/L (previous 0.8). Management included:

- Holding lithium temporarily
- IV hydration
- Switching to verapamil for migraine prevention
- Using NSAIDs cautiously for headaches

- Coordinating care between specialists

This case emphasizes how interactions extend beyond direct drug-drug effects to include masking of toxicity symptoms and altered monitoring parameters.

## Building Systematic Safety

Drug interaction prevention requires systematic approaches rather than perfect memory. Key strategies include:

1. **Maintain complete medication lists** including OTC drugs and supplements
2. **Use interaction checkers** but interpret results clinically
3. **Communicate between prescribers** especially specialists
4. **Educate patients** about interaction risks and symptoms
5. **Monitor appropriately** based on interaction potential
6. **Start low, go slow** when adding medications
7. **Document interaction checks** in clinical notes

Understanding basic principles—which drugs inhibit or induce which enzymes, which combinations increase serotonin, which prolong QT—provides a framework for safe prescribing. Perfect knowledge isn't required; systematic checking and clinical vigilance prevent most serious interactions.

### Key Takeaways

- The CYP450 system functions like a highway system where drugs compete for metabolism
- CYP3A4 processes over 50% of medications while CYP2D6 handles many psychiatric drugs
- Strong inhibitors like fluoxetine can double or triple levels of other medications
- Serotonin syndrome presents with mental status changes, autonomic dysfunction, and neuromuscular abnormalities
- Early recognition and stopping serotonergic drugs immediately improves outcomes

- QT prolongation risk increases with multiple medications, electrolyte abnormalities, and cardiac disease
- Systematic interaction checking at each medication change prevents most serious events
- Communication between prescribers reduces dangerous combinations
- Natural supplements can cause serious interactions with psychiatric medications
- Clinical judgment must interpret interaction warnings in context of individual patients

# Chapter 10: Special Populations in Detail

Treating psychiatric conditions in special populations requires adjusting standard approaches to account for unique physiological states, developmental considerations, and increased vulnerabilities. Pregnancy transforms medication decisions into complex risk-benefit calculations affecting two lives. Children's developing brains respond unpredictably to psychiatric medications. Elderly patients' declining organ function and multiple medications create fragility requiring careful management. Understanding these populations' specific needs prevents harm while ensuring necessary treatment continues.

## Pregnancy and Breastfeeding

The discovery of pregnancy in a woman taking psychiatric medications creates immediate anxiety for patients and clinicians alike. Years of "pregnancy category" warnings trained everyone to fear medications during pregnancy, yet untreated mental illness poses its own serious risks. Modern understanding emphasizes individualized risk-benefit discussions rather than blanket medication discontinuation.

**Risk-benefit discussions made simple** start with acknowledging that no decision carries zero risk. The question becomes: which option poses less risk—continuing medication or stopping it? This requires understanding both medication risks and illness risks.

Untreated mental illness during pregnancy associates with:

- Increased preterm birth and low birth weight
- Poor prenatal care and nutrition
- Substance use as self-medication
- Suicide (leading cause of maternal mortality)
- Impaired bonding and parenting
- Relationship disruption
- Job loss and financial stress

Medication risks vary by timing:

- First trimester: organ formation (teratogenesis risk)
- Second trimester: growth and development
- Third trimester: neonatal adaptation syndromes
- Throughout: potential neurodevelopmental effects

The key message: psychiatric stability benefits both mother and baby. Most women with moderate to severe mental illness should continue treatment with appropriate monitoring (126).

**Medication selection guidelines** prioritize older medications with more safety data over newer options:

**Antidepressants**: SSRIs remain first-line with extensive reassuring data. Sertraline shows lowest placental transfer. Paroxetine carries slightly higher cardiac malformation risk but remains reasonable if patient stable. SNRIs appear similarly safe. Avoid paroxetine in first trimester if possible.

**Mood stabilizers**: Lithium carries 0.05-0.1% risk of Ebstein's anomaly (cardiac defect) versus 0.01% baseline—increased but still rare. Lamotrigine shows good safety data. Valproic acid causes neural tube defects in 1-2% and decreased IQ—avoid entirely. Carbamazepine also increases neural tube defects.

**Antipsychotics**: Older antipsychotics have more data suggesting relative safety. Haloperidol shows extensive safe use. Second-generation antipsychotics appear similarly safe with growing data. Monitor for gestational diabetes with metabolic effects.

**Benzodiazepines**: Older studies suggested cleft palate risk, but newer data shows minimal increase. Greater concern involves "floppy baby syndrome" with third-trimester use. Use lowest doses for shortest duration.

**Monitoring mom and baby** requires collaborative care between psychiatry, obstetrics, and pediatrics:

Maternal monitoring:

95

- Monthly psychiatric visits minimum
- Increase frequency in third trimester
- Monitor blood levels (may need dose adjustments)
- Screen for gestational diabetes with antipsychotics
- Watch for postpartum mood episodes

Fetal monitoring:

- Level II ultrasound at 18-20 weeks
- Fetal echocardiography with lithium
- Growth scans with medications affecting weight
- Non-stress tests if concerns arise

Neonatal planning:

- Inform pediatrics about medications
- Plan for possible NICU observation
- Watch for withdrawal or toxicity symptoms
- Support breastfeeding decisions

## Case Study: Managing Bipolar Disorder in Pregnancy

Rachel, 31, had severe bipolar I disorder well-controlled on lithium 900 mg and quetiapine 200 mg. She presented 6 weeks pregnant (unplanned but wanted pregnancy) terrified about medications harming her baby. "Should I stop everything?" she asked anxiously.

History revealed:

- Two previous manic episodes requiring hospitalization
- One postpartum psychosis with first child
- Stable on current regimen for 3 years
- Strong family support
- No substance use

Risk-benefit discussion covered:

- High risk of relapse if medications stopped

96

- Previous postpartum psychosis increases recurrence risk to 50%
- Lithium's small absolute risk of cardiac defects
- Quetiapine's reassuring safety data
- Risks of mania during pregnancy

Collaborative decision:

- Continue both medications with close monitoring
- Lithium levels monthly (increased renal clearance requires dose adjustments)
- Fetal echocardiography at 20 weeks
- Coordinate with high-risk obstetrics
- Plan for postpartum monitoring

Management through pregnancy:

- First trimester: Lithium increased to 1200 mg for therapeutic levels
- Second trimester: Stable with monthly monitoring
- Third trimester: Lithium reduced to avoid neonatal toxicity
- Delivery: Psychiatry consulted for immediate postpartum management

Outcome:

- Healthy baby girl, brief NICU observation for mild tremor
- Rachel remained stable throughout pregnancy
- Immediate lithium restart postpartum prevented mood episode
- Successful breastfeeding with careful medication selection

This case illustrates how thoughtful risk-benefit analysis and collaborative care enables successful outcomes.

## Children and Adolescents

Pediatric psychopharmacology requires acknowledging fundamental differences from adult treatment. Children aren't simply small adults—their developing brains respond differently to medications, creating unique benefits and risks requiring specialized knowledge.

**Black box warnings explained** create fear but require context. The FDA black box warning states antidepressants increase suicidal thinking and behavior in children and adolescents. The numbers: roughly 4% with antidepressants versus 2% with placebo showed increased suicidal ideation. No completed suicides occurred in trials.

However, context matters:

- Untreated depression carries 15% lifetime suicide risk
- Adolescent suicide rates decreased as SSRI use increased
- Benefits outweigh risks for moderate-severe depression
- Close monitoring catches problems early

The warning's purpose: ensure proper monitoring, not prevent treatment. Think of it like seatbelt warnings—they can cause injuries in crashes, but overall save lives (127).

**Dosing considerations** in youth reflect both pharmacokinetic and pharmacodynamic differences:

Pharmacokinetic differences:

- Faster metabolism requires higher mg/kg doses
- Shorter half-lives may need divided dosing
- Variable absorption affects blood levels
- Less protein binding increases free drug

Pharmacodynamic differences:

- Developing receptors show different sensitivities
- Increased activation and behavioral disinhibition
- Paradoxical reactions more common
- Side effects may differ from adults

Practical dosing approach:

- Start lower than adult doses initially
- Titrate based on response, not mg/kg calculations
- May eventually need adult or higher doses
- Monitor closely during dose changes

**Family involvement strategies** recognize that pediatric treatment succeeds only with family engagement:

Education priorities:

- Explain black box warning accurately
- Discuss realistic timeline (6-8 weeks for full effect)
- Review common side effects
- Create monitoring plan together
- Emphasize adherence importance

Monitoring assignments:

- Parents observe for behavior changes
- Teachers report academic/social functioning
- Patient uses mood tracking apps
- Regular check-ins first month
- Clear emergency contact plan

Communication strategies:

- Include adolescents in discussions appropriately
- Respect developing autonomy
- Address family medication fears
- Cultural sensitivity essential
- Written materials reinforce verbal education

## Case Example 1: The Activated Adolescent

Tyler, 14, started fluoxetine 10 mg for severe depression and anxiety. After two weeks, his mother called urgently: "He's not sleeping, talking nonstop, and got in three fights at school. He's never been like this."

Assessment revealed:

- Sleeping 2-3 hours nightly
- Excessive energy and goal-directed activity
- Irritability and aggression
- No previous manic symptoms
- Family history significant for bipolar disorder

This represented antidepressant-induced mania, not simple activation. Management:

- Stopped fluoxetine immediately
- Started lithium for mood stabilization
- Brief course of risperidone for acute mania
- Revised diagnosis to bipolar disorder

Tyler's case illustrates how antidepressants can unmask bipolar disorder in youth, requiring vigilant monitoring for activation beyond anxiety.

## Geriatric Considerations

Aging transforms medication management through multiple mechanisms: decreased kidney and liver function slow drug clearance, altered body composition affects drug distribution, increased brain sensitivity magnifies effects, and polypharmacy multiplies interaction risks. These changes demand modified approaches summarized by "start low, go slow—but go."

**Beers Criteria simplified** provides guidance on potentially inappropriate medications in elderly patients. Think of it as a caution list rather than absolute contraindications—clinical judgment weighs risks against benefits.

Key psychiatric medications on Beers Criteria:

- Benzodiazepines: increase falls, cognitive impairment
- Tertiary TCAs (amitriptyline): anticholinergic effects

- Antipsychotics: stroke risk in dementia
- Z-drugs: similar risks to benzodiazepines
- Paroxetine: most anticholinergic SSRI

Safer alternatives in elderly:

- SSRIs: sertraline, citalopram (max 20 mg), escitalopram
- SNRIs: duloxetine (helpful for pain)
- Bupropion: if activation tolerated
- Mirtazapine: helps sleep and appetite
- Buspirone: anxiety without sedation

The key: avoiding medications doesn't mean avoiding treatment. Choose safer alternatives and monitor closely (128).

**Polypharmacy management** addresses the average elderly patient taking 5-9 medications. Each additional medication exponentially increases adverse event risk. Strategies include:

Systematic review:

- List all medications including OTC
- Identify duplications (multiple anticholinergics)
- Check for drug-drug interactions
- Assess ongoing need for each medication
- Consider deprescribing stable patients

Coordination approaches:

- Single pharmacy for all medications
- Medication reconciliation at each visit
- Brown bag reviews periodically
- Coordinate with all prescribers
- Simplify regimens when possible

**Fall risk reduction** recognizes falls as a leading cause of morbidity in elderly. Psychiatric medications particularly increase risk through sedation, orthostatic hypotension, and cognitive effects (129).

Fall risk medications:

- Benzodiazepines (highest risk)
- Sedating antidepressants (TCAs, mirtazapine)
- Antipsychotics
- Multiple CNS-active medications

Risk reduction strategies:

- Use lowest effective doses
- Avoid multiple sedating medications
- Check orthostatic blood pressure
- Time sedating medications at bedtime
- Physical therapy referral
- Home safety evaluation
- Vitamin D supplementation

## Case Example 2: The Complex Elderly Patient

Dorothy, 78, presented with depression following her husband's death. Her medications included:

- Amitriptyline 100 mg for decades ("the only thing that helps")
- Lorazepam 1 mg three times daily for anxiety
- Zolpidem 10 mg for sleep
- Gabapentin 300 mg for neuropathy
- Multiple cardiac medications

She reported three falls in two months, memory problems, and constipation.

This represented a geriatric medication disaster. Approach:

1. Build trust—acknowledge amitriptyline helped historically
2. Explain how aging changed medication effects
3. Propose gradual transitions, not abrupt changes

Medication adjustments over 3 months:

- Switched amitriptyline to nortriptyline 50 mg (less anticholinergic)
- Tapered lorazepam using longer-acting clonazepam
- Discontinued zolpidem, used melatonin
- Eventually transitioned to sertraline
- Maintained gabapentin for pain

Outcomes:

- No falls in 6 months
- Improved cognition
- Resolved constipation
- Maintained mood stability

This case shows how careful deprescribing and switching to safer alternatives improves outcomes without sacrificing efficacy.

## Case Example 3: The Pregnant Professional

Amanda, 35, a physician herself, took venlafaxine 225 mg for severe anxiety and depression. She presented 5 weeks pregnant after years of infertility treatment. "I know I should stop the medication," she stated, "but I'm terrified of relapsing during pregnancy."

Her history revealed:

- Two previous severe depressive episodes
- One suicide attempt in medical school
- Excellent response to venlafaxine after failing SSRIs
- High-stress job requiring cognitive function
- Strong desire for healthy pregnancy

Risk-benefit discussion challenged her assumptions:

- Venlafaxine shows reassuring pregnancy data
- Her severe depression history posed significant risks
- Physician suicide risk remains elevated
- Stress hormones affect fetal development

- Stable mothers have better pregnancy outcomes

Collaborative plan:

- Continue venlafaxine with close monitoring
- Increased therapy frequency
- Coordinate with maternal-fetal medicine
- Plan for postpartum support
- Address perfectionism and control issues

Amanda initially resisted continuing medication but agreed after thorough discussion. She remained stable throughout pregnancy, delivered a healthy baby, and successfully breastfed while continuing venlafaxine.

"My colleagues judged me for taking medication while pregnant," she reflected, "but I couldn't care for my baby if I were severely depressed. That discussion saved both our lives."

## Adapting Treatment for Success

Special populations require modified approaches, not medication avoidance. Pregnancy demands careful risk-benefit analysis balancing maternal mental health against fetal exposure. Children need close monitoring for unique responses while involving families in treatment. Elderly patients benefit from "geriatric-friendly" medications and systematic deprescribing of harmful drugs.

Success requires patience, flexibility, and recognition that one-size-fits-all approaches fail these vulnerable populations. By understanding their unique needs and adjusting treatment accordingly, clinicians can provide safe, effective care throughout the lifespan.

### Key Takeaways

- Untreated mental illness during pregnancy poses significant risks to both mother and baby

- Most psychiatric medications show reassuring safety data with appropriate monitoring
- Older medications with extensive data are preferred during pregnancy over newer options
- Black box warnings for adolescents require perspective—benefits outweigh risks for moderate-severe depression
- Children metabolize medications faster but show increased behavioral sensitivity
- Family involvement is essential for successful pediatric treatment
- Beers Criteria guides but doesn't dictate elderly medication choices
- Polypharmacy exponentially increases adverse events in elderly patients
- Fall prevention requires systematic assessment of sedating medications
- Success in special populations requires individualized risk-benefit analysis rather than rigid rules

# Chapter 11: Practical Clinical Scenarios

Real-world psychiatric practice rarely presents textbook cases. Patients arrive with multiple diagnoses, failed medication trials, cultural considerations, and complex psychosocial situations that challenge standard approaches. These practical scenarios illustrate how to navigate common clinical complexities while maintaining safety and therapeutic relationships.

## Treatment-Resistant Depression: Step-by-Step Approaches

Treatment-resistant depression (TRD) affects 30% of patients with major depression, defined as failure to respond to two adequate antidepressant trials. However, many "treatment-resistant" cases actually represent inadequate trials, missed diagnoses, or unaddressed contributing factors. Systematic evaluation often reveals correctable problems.

### Step 1: Verify True Treatment Resistance

- Confirm adequate dose and duration (minimum 6-8 weeks at therapeutic dose)
- Assess adherence through pharmacy records and blood levels
- Screen for bipolar disorder (antidepressants alone worsen bipolar depression)
- Identify substance use (alcohol negates antidepressant effects)
- Check thyroid function (subclinical hypothyroidism impairs response)
- Evaluate sleep disorders (untreated sleep apnea prevents improvement)

### Step 2: Optimize Current Treatment

- Increase dose to maximum tolerated
- Add psychotherapy if not already present
- Address psychosocial stressors

- Treat comorbid anxiety (residual anxiety predicts poor response)
- Optimize general health (exercise, nutrition, sleep hygiene)

**Step 3: Augmentation Strategies** First-line augmentation:

- Aripiprazole 2-10 mg (FDA approved)
- Lithium 600-900 mg (extensive evidence)
- T3 thyroid hormone 25-50 mcg
- Buspirone 30-60 mg divided

Second-line options:

- Quetiapine 150-300 mg
- Lamotrigine 100-200 mg
- Methylfolate 15 mg (especially with MTHFR mutations)
- Omega-3 fatty acids 2-4 grams

**Step 4: Switching Strategies**

- Switch to different class (SSRI to SNRI or vice versa)
- Try medications with unique mechanisms (bupropion, mirtazapine)
- Consider MAOIs for patients failing multiple trials
- Evaluate ketamine/esketamine for rapid response needs

**Step 5: Combination Antidepressants**

- SSRI/SNRI + mirtazapine ("California rocket fuel")
- SSRI + bupropion (addresses multiple neurotransmitters)
- Venlafaxine + mirtazapine (powerful but monitor for serotonin syndrome)

**Step 6: Novel Approaches**

- Transcranial magnetic stimulation (TMS)
- Electroconvulsive therapy (ECT) for severe cases
- Vagus nerve stimulation
- Deep brain stimulation (experimental)

- Psychedelic-assisted therapy (emerging evidence) (130)

## Case Example 1: Breaking Through Resistance

James, 52, tried six antidepressants over three years without significant improvement. Review revealed:

- "Adequate" trials were actually 4 weeks at subtherapeutic doses
- Untreated sleep apnea caused severe fatigue
- Daily marijuana use for "medical purposes"
- Subclinical hypothyroidism (TSH 4.8)

Systematic approach:

1. Started CPAP for sleep apnea
2. Added levothyroxine for thyroid optimization
3. Addressed marijuana use through motivational interviewing
4. Retried sertraline at 200 mg for 8 weeks
5. Added aripiprazole 5 mg when partial response achieved

Within 3 months, James achieved remission for the first time. "I wasn't really treatment-resistant," he reflected. "We just hadn't addressed the whole picture."

## Managing Non-adherence: Real-World Strategies

Medication non-adherence affects 50% of psychiatric patients, driven by side effects, lack of insight, cost, complexity, and stigma. Lecturing about adherence fails—understanding individual barriers and collaborative problem-solving succeeds.

### Common adherence barriers and solutions:

Side effects:

- Take detailed side effect history
- Adjust timing, dose, or formulation

- Add medications to counter side effects
- Switch to better-tolerated alternatives
- Set realistic expectations about timeline

Cost:

- Prescribe generics when possible
- Use patient assistance programs
- Provide samples for bridges
- Simplify regimens to reduce pill burden
- Split higher-dose tablets when appropriate

Complexity:

- Use pill organizers or blister packs
- Recommend medication reminder apps
- Prescribe long-acting formulations
- Combine medications when possible
- Create written schedules with pictures

Stigma:

- Normalize medication use
- Address cultural beliefs respectfully
- Involve trusted family members
- Reframe as "vitamins for the brain"
- Focus on functional improvements

Lack of insight:

- Use motivational interviewing techniques
- Focus on patient-identified goals
- Track objective improvements
- Involve family observations
- Consider long-acting injectables (131)

**Practical adherence interventions:**

"Forgetting" medications:

- Link to established routines (brushing teeth)
- Use smartphone alarms with specific labels
- Place medications in visible locations
- Consider automatic dispensers
- Weekly pill organization sessions

"They don't work":

- Review timeline expectations
- Track specific symptoms objectively
- Identify partial improvements patient missed
- Address all-or-nothing thinking
- Adjust doses before abandoning

"I feel better and don't need them":

- Educate about maintenance treatment
- Use diabetes/hypertension analogies
- Review past relapses
- Create written relapse prevention plans
- Schedule regular check-ins

## Case Example 2: The Ambivalent Patient

Maria, 38, repeatedly stopped her bipolar medications despite multiple hospitalizations. Exploration revealed:

- Medications reminded her she was "broken"
- Weight gain affected self-esteem
- Husband said she was "more fun" when manic
- Cost stressed limited budget
- Complex regimen felt overwhelming

Collaborative solutions:

1. Reframed medications as tools for achieving her goals
2. Switched to weight-neutral options (lithium to lamotrigine)
3. Included husband in education about mania's destruction

4. Applied for patient assistance programs
5. Simplified to once-daily regimen
6. Created personal "reasons to take medication" list

Maria's adherence improved dramatically when barriers were addressed individually rather than generically.

## Emergency Situations: Office-Based Responses

Psychiatric emergencies in outpatient settings require rapid assessment and decisive action while maintaining safety for all involved. Preparation and clear protocols prevent panic when crises arise.

**Acute suicidality protocol:**

1. Direct assessment: "Are you thinking of killing yourself?"
2. Determine immediacy: plan, means, intent, timeline
3. Remove means if possible (medications, weapons)
4. Never leave actively suicidal patient alone
5. Involve support system immediately
6. Determine appropriate level of care:
   o Safety plan for low risk
   o Emergency evaluation for moderate risk
   o Direct transport to ED for high risk
7. Document thoroughly including rationale
8. Follow up within 24-48 hours

**Severe agitation management:**

1. Ensure staff safety first
2. Use calm, non-threatening approach
3. Offer voluntary medication (oral preferred)
4. Set clear limits and consequences
5. Call security/police if violence imminent
6. Document precipitants and interventions
7. Debrief with patient when calm

**Acute medication reactions:**

1. Stop suspected medication immediately
2. Assess vital signs if possible
3. Call 911 for severe symptoms
4. Provide medication list to EMS
5. Contact prescriber urgently
6. Document timeline and symptoms
7. Follow up after emergency treatment

## Complex Cases: Multiple Diagnoses, Multiple Medications

Real-world patients rarely have single, uncomplicated diagnoses. Comorbidity represents the rule rather than exception, requiring thoughtful prioritization and systematic management.

**Principles for complex cases:**

1. Establish diagnostic hierarchy
2. Treat most severe/dangerous condition first
3. Use medications addressing multiple conditions
4. Monitor for drug interactions vigilantly
5. Simplify regimens whenever possible
6. Coordinate care among providers
7. Set realistic expectations

**Common comorbidity patterns:**

Depression + Anxiety:

- SSRIs/SNRIs address both conditions
- Avoid benzodiazepines if possible
- Add buspirone for residual anxiety
- Consider mirtazapine for sleep issues

Bipolar + ADHD:

- Stabilize mood before treating ADHD

- Use non-stimulants when possible
- Monitor carefully for mania with stimulants
- Consider atomoxetine or bupropion

Psychosis + Substance Use:

- Choose antipsychotics with lower abuse potential
- Avoid benzodiazepines if possible
- Use long-acting injectables for adherence
- Integrate addiction treatment

PTSD + Chronic Pain:

- SNRIs address both conditions
- Avoid benzodiazepines and opioids together
- Consider prazosin for nightmares
- Add gabapentin for neuropathic pain

## Case Example 3: The Complex Case Conference

Robert, 45, presented with:

- Bipolar I disorder
- PTSD from combat trauma
- Alcohol use disorder (early recovery)
- Chronic back pain
- Hypertension
- Obesity

Current medications:

- Lithium 900 mg (mood stabilizer)
- Quetiapine 400 mg (mood/sleep)
- Prazosin 5 mg (nightmares)
- Gabapentin 800 mg TID (pain/anxiety)
- Lisinopril 20 mg (blood pressure)
- Naltrexone 50 mg (alcohol cravings)

Problems identified:

- 40-pound weight gain from quetiapine
- Sedation affecting work
- Breakthrough mood symptoms
- Continued pain limiting function
- Poor adherence due to complexity

Systematic approach:

1. Prioritized mood stability and sobriety
2. Switched quetiapine to lurasidone (weight-neutral)
3. Added lamotrigine for mood stabilization
4. Optimized gabapentin dosing for pain
5. Referred to weight management program
6. Simplified dosing to twice daily maximum
7. Coordinated with all providers

Six months later: 20-pound weight loss, improved mood stability, sustained sobriety, and better adherence with simplified regimen.

## Cultural Considerations: Adapting Approaches

Cultural factors profoundly influence medication attitudes, adherence, and response. Effective treatment requires cultural humility and willingness to adapt Western medical approaches to diverse belief systems.

**Key cultural factors affecting medication treatment:**

Beliefs about mental illness:

- Spiritual/religious explanations
- Stigma and shame
- Family versus individual focus
- Mind-body integration concepts
- Traditional healing practices

Medication attitudes:

- "Natural" versus "chemical" preferences
- Fear of dependence/addiction
- Concern about personality changes
- Trust in medical systems
- Previous cultural traumas

Communication styles:

- Direct versus indirect
- Family involvement expectations
- Authority relationships
- Emotional expression norms
- Language barriers

**Practical cultural adaptations:**

Asian populations:

- Start with lower doses (genetic variations)
- Address stigma through medical model
- Involve family with permission
- Respect complementary treatments
- Monitor closely for side effects

Hispanic/Latino populations:

- Use "nervios" or culturally relevant terms
- Address religious concerns
- Include extended family
- Respect traditional remedies
- Consider language-concordant providers

African American populations:

- Acknowledge historical medical mistrust
- Discuss concerns openly
- Start conservatively with antipsychotics

- Address spiritual frameworks
- Ensure culturally competent providers

Native American populations:

- Respect traditional healing
- Avoid rushing treatment decisions
- Include tribal healers if desired
- Address historical trauma
- Consider cultural concepts of wellness (132)

## Integrating All Elements

Complex clinical scenarios require integrating multiple skills: diagnostic accuracy, medication knowledge, cultural competence, and relationship building. Success comes from systematic approaches adapted to individual circumstances rather than rigid protocols.

The art lies in balancing evidence-based medicine with person-centered care. What works in research studies may need modification for the patient sitting in front of you with their unique constellation of diagnoses, life circumstances, and cultural background.

By mastering these practical scenarios, clinicians develop confidence handling the messy realities of psychiatric practice. Perfect outcomes remain rare, but thoughtful, systematic approaches improve results while maintaining therapeutic relationships through challenges.

### Key Takeaways

- True treatment-resistant depression is rare—most cases represent inadequate trials or missed contributing factors
- Systematic augmentation and switching strategies help patients who don't respond to initial treatments
- Medication adherence improves when individual barriers are addressed collaboratively
- Emergency situations require clear protocols and decisive action while maintaining safety

- Complex comorbidities benefit from medications addressing multiple conditions simultaneously
- Cultural factors profoundly influence medication attitudes requiring adapted approaches
- Success with challenging cases comes from systematic yet flexible patient-centered care
- Documentation of complex decision-making protects both patients and clinicians
- Coordinated care among multiple providers prevents dangerous interactions and improves outcomes
- Realistic expectations and strong therapeutic relationships sustain treatment through difficulties

As psychopharmacology continues advancing rapidly, with new mechanisms, delivery methods, and precision medicine approaches emerging. Yet the fundamentals remain constant: careful assessment, thoughtful medication selection, vigilant monitoring, and strong therapeutic relationships drive successful outcomes.

As you apply these concepts in practice, remember that medication represents just one tool in comprehensive mental health treatment. The goal isn't perfect pharmacology but helping patients build meaningful, functional lives. Sometimes that means accepting partial improvement rather than risking destabilization chasing perfection. Other times it requires taking calculated risks with novel approaches when standard treatments fail.

Your growth as a clinician comes from each challenging case, each creative solution, and each lesson learned from both successes and failures. Keep learning, stay curious, and maintain hope—for in mental health treatment, transformation remains possible even in the most complex situations.

# Chapter 12: Essential References

Clinical practice demands quick access to accurate information during busy days filled with complex decisions. While memorizing every medication detail remains impossible, having well-organized reference materials transforms overwhelming pharmacology into manageable clinical tools. This chapter provides practical resources you'll actually use—not theoretical knowledge that sounds impressive but fails in real-world application. These references live on your desk, phone, or clipboard, ready when you need specific doses, monitoring schedules, or emergency guidance.

## Medication Comparison Tables

Understanding medication differences at a glance saves precious time and prevents errors. Rather than flipping through multiple resources or relying on memory, these comparisons highlight key distinctions that guide clinical decisions.

**Antidepressants at a glance** reveals patterns that inform selection:

SSRIs share similar efficacy but differ in practical ways. Fluoxetine's 4-6 day half-life provides built-in protection against withdrawal but means side effects linger. Starting doses range from 10-20 mg daily, increasing to 40-80 mg for full effect. Its active metabolite and CYP2D6 inhibition create complex interactions lasting weeks after discontinuation.

Sertraline offers the middle ground—25-50 mg starting dose, titrating to 100-200 mg daily. Minimal drug interactions and balanced side effects make it many clinicians' first choice. The shorter half-life than fluoxetine allows quicker adjustments but requires consistent daily dosing.

Paroxetine starts at 10-20 mg, increasing to 40-60 mg, but causes more anticholinergic effects, weight gain, and sexual dysfunction than other SSRIs. Its short half-life creates severe withdrawal symptoms with missed doses. Many clinicians avoid it except when sedation helps anxious patients.

Escitalopram begins at 5-10 mg daily, maxing at 20 mg (10 mg if over 60 or with CYP2C19 inhibitors). As the refined version of citalopram, it causes fewer side effects at equivalent doses. Minimal drug interactions make it suitable for complex patients.

SNRIs add norepinephrine effects that help energy and pain. Venlafaxine immediate-release starts at 37.5 mg twice daily, extended-release at 75 mg once daily, titrating to 225-375 mg. Blood pressure monitoring becomes essential above 225 mg. Severe withdrawal symptoms require extremely gradual tapering.

Duloxetine begins at 30 mg daily, increasing to 60-120 mg. FDA approvals for multiple pain conditions make it logical when depression coexists with fibromyalgia or neuropathy. The capsule can't be opened or crushed, limiting flexibility.

Atypical antidepressants fill specific niches. Bupropion starts at 150 mg daily, increasing to 300-450 mg divided or extended-release. No sexual side effects and potential weight loss benefit many patients, but seizure risk requires screening. Avoid doses above 450 mg daily or 200 mg at once with immediate-release.

Mirtazapine's dosing paradox confuses many—7.5-15 mg causes more sedation than 30-45 mg due to emerging norepinephrine effects at higher doses. Weight gain and sedation limit use but help depressed patients with insomnia and poor appetite.

**Mood stabilizer monitoring requirements** prevent serious complications:

Lithium demands the most intensive monitoring. Baseline labs include CBC, electrolytes, creatinine, TSH, and EKG if over 50. Check levels weekly during initiation, then monthly for three months, then every 3-6 months indefinitely. Draw levels 12 hours post-dose for accuracy. Monitor creatinine and TSH every 6 months long-term.

Target levels: 0.6-1.2 mEq/L for maintenance, sometimes higher for acute mania.

Valproic acid requires baseline CBC, liver function, and pregnancy test for women. Check levels 5 days after changes, then every 3-6 months. Monitor CBC and liver function every 6 months. Women need ongoing pregnancy prevention counseling. Target levels: 50-125 μg/mL, though some respond outside this range.

Lamotrigine needs minimal lab monitoring—mainly watching for rash during titration. No therapeutic levels guide dosing. The critical slow titration prevents Stevens-Johnson syndrome: 25 mg daily for 2 weeks, 50 mg for 2 weeks, then 50 mg increases every 2 weeks to 200 mg. With valproic acid, start 25 mg every other day due to doubled levels.

Carbamazepine requires baseline CBC and liver function, then frequent monitoring initially due to blood dyscrasia risk. Check levels, CBC, and liver function at 2 weeks, 1 month, then every 3-6 months. Watch for dropping levels due to auto-induction. Multiple drug interactions necessitate careful monitoring with any medication changes. Target levels: 4-12 μg/mL.

**Antipsychotic metabolic risk stratification** guides monitoring intensity:

High metabolic risk medications (clozapine, olanzapine) cause severe weight gain and diabetes risk. Average weight gain exceeds 10 kg. Monitor weight monthly for 3 months, then quarterly. Check glucose and lipids at baseline, 3 months, then every 6 months. Consider prophylactic metformin for high-risk patients.

Moderate risk drugs (quetiapine, risperidone, paliperidone) typically cause 3-5 kg weight gain. Monitor weight and blood pressure monthly initially, then quarterly. Metabolic labs at baseline, 3 months, annually thereafter. Switch medications if weight gain exceeds 7% body weight.

Lower risk options (aripiprazole, ziprasidone, lurasidone) minimize metabolic effects but aren't risk-free. Monitor weight quarterly, metabolic labs annually. These represent first choices for patients with diabetes or metabolic syndrome. Ziprasidone requires EKG monitoring due to QT prolongation.

**Anxiolytic duration and potency** determines clinical use:

Ultra-short acting: Triazolam works within 15-30 minutes, lasting 2-3 hours. Reserve for sleep initiation only. High abuse potential and anterograde amnesia risk limit use.

Short-acting: Alprazolam onset 30-60 minutes, duration 6-12 hours. Requires multiple daily doses for sustained anxiety control. Severe rebound anxiety and withdrawal with short half-life. Lorazepam onset 1-2 hours, duration 12-20 hours, with more reliable absorption than other benzodiazepines.

Intermediate-acting: Temazepam primarily for insomnia, onset 30-60 minutes, duration 8-12 hours. Less abuse potential than ultra-short agents.

Long-acting: Clonazepam onset 1-4 hours, duration 18-50 hours. Once or twice daily dosing improves adherence. Less rebound anxiety between doses. Diazepam rapid onset within 30 minutes, very long half-life (20-100 hours) accumulates in elderly. Active metabolites extend duration.

## Case Example 1: The Confusing Consultation

Dr. Martinez called about a shared patient: "Mrs. Chen is on some antidepressant—I think Lexapro? Maybe Cymbalta? She needs surgery next month. Any concerns with anesthesia?"

Without clear documentation, determining interaction risks becomes impossible. Quick reference confirmed:

- Escitalopram (Lexapro): Minimal anesthesia interactions, mild bleeding risk with NSAIDs
- Duloxetine (Cymbalta): Inhibits CYP2D6, affecting some anesthetics; bleeding risk higher

Phone call back to confirm medication revealed duloxetine 60 mg. Guidance provided:

- Continue through surgery (withdrawal risk exceeds bleeding risk)
- Alert anesthesia about CYP2D6 inhibition
- Avoid tramadol post-operatively (serotonin syndrome risk)
- Monitor for increased bleeding

This case demonstrates how quick access to comparison data enables accurate consultation responses.

## Dosing Quick Guides

Starting psychiatric medications requires balancing efficacy needs against tolerability. These guides provide evidence-based starting points adapted to specific populations and situations.

**Starting doses for common scenarios** vary by patient factors:

Healthy adults typically tolerate standard starting doses. Begin SSRIs at lower therapeutic doses: sertraline 50 mg, escitalopram 10 mg, fluoxetine 20 mg. SNRIs start similarly: duloxetine 30 mg, venlafaxine XR 75 mg. Anxiety may temporarily worsen before improving—warn patients to prevent early discontinuation.

Elderly patients need "geriatric dosing"—typically half standard adult doses. Start sertraline 25 mg, escitalopram 5 mg, duloxetine 20 mg. Even with dose adjustments, monitor closely for falls, hyponatremia, and cognitive effects. The principle "start low, go slow" prevents adverse events while still treating effectively.

Anxious patients benefit from extra-cautious initiation. Consider starting at pediatric doses: sertraline 12.5 mg, escitalopram 2.5 mg (liquid formulation). Explain that physical anxiety symptoms may increase initially. Some clinicians add short-term benzodiazepines during initiation, though this requires careful monitoring.

Medically complex patients with multiple conditions need individualized approaches. Reduce doses with hepatic impairment (most psychiatric medications undergo liver metabolism). Renal impairment affects lithium, gabapentin, and pregabalin primarily. Drug interactions may necessitate lower starting doses—check interactions before initiating.

**Titration schedules** balance speed against tolerability:

SSRIs typically increase every 1-2 weeks. After starting sertraline 50 mg, increase by 25-50 mg increments to maximum 200 mg. Escitalopram increases by 5 mg increments to maximum 20 mg (10 mg in elderly). Allow 4-6 weeks at target dose before assessing response.

SNRIs require similar patience. Venlafaxine XR increases by 75 mg every 4-7 days to target 150-225 mg. Some patients need 300-375 mg for full response. Monitor blood pressure with doses above 225 mg. Duloxetine typically increases from 30 mg to 60 mg after one week, with some patients needing 90-120 mg.

Mood stabilizers demand variable approaches. Lithium starts at 300 mg once or twice daily, increasing by 300 mg every 3-5 days based on levels and tolerance. Lamotrigine requires rigid adherence to slow titration preventing dangerous rashes. Valproic acid can load at 20 mg/kg for acute mania or start at 250 mg twice daily for maintenance.

Antipsychotics titrate based on indication. For acute psychosis, reach therapeutic doses quickly—risperidone 2-4 mg, olanzapine 10-20 mg within days. For depression augmentation or anxiety, start lower and increase slowly—aripiprazole 2 mg, quetiapine 25-50 mg.

**Maximum recommended doses** prevent toxicity while recognizing some patients need higher amounts:

FDA maximum doses provide safety guidelines but aren't absolute ceilings. Fluoxetine's maximum 80 mg daily suffices for most patients, though some require 100-120 mg with careful monitoring. Sertraline maxes at 200 mg but occasional patients benefit from 250-300 mg, particularly for OCD.

Higher than FDA doses require documentation of:

- Failed adequate trials at standard doses
- Partial response suggesting more might help
- Absence of limiting side effects
- Patient consent to off-label dosing
- Plan for increased monitoring

Some maximums reflect safety concerns rather than efficacy plateaus. Citalopram's 40 mg limit (20 mg in elderly) prevents QT prolongation. Bupropion's 450 mg maximum reduces seizure risk. These represent firmer ceilings than efficacy-based limits.

## Monitoring Checklists

Systematic monitoring catches problems before they become serious while avoiding excessive testing that burdens patients without benefit. These checklists ensure nothing falls through cracks during busy clinical practice.

**Laboratory schedules** vary by medication class:

Lithium monitoring remains most intensive:

- Baseline: CBC, BUN/creatinine, TSH, electrolytes, EKG if >50
- Weekly levels during initiation
- Monthly levels and creatinine for 3 months
- Every 3-6 months: level, creatinine, TSH

- Annual: CBC, electrolytes, calcium

Antipsychotic monitoring focuses on metabolic effects:

- Baseline: Weight, waist circumference, BP, fasting glucose, lipids
- Monthly weights for 3 months
- 3 months: Repeat all baseline measures
- Every 6 months first year: glucose, lipids
- Annually thereafter if stable
- More frequent monitoring with significant weight gain

Antidepressant monitoring stays minimal:

- Baseline: Consider EKG with tricyclics or citalopram
- Sodium check at 2-4 weeks in elderly (SIADH risk)
- Otherwise monitoring focuses on clinical response
- Annual metabolic labs reasonable with weight gain

**Clinical assessment timelines** ensure systematic evaluation:

Week 1-2: Contact high-risk patients (elderly, adolescents, complex cases). Assess tolerability, early side effects, and adherence. Address misconceptions before they lead to discontinuation.

Week 4: Full assessment including side effects, partial response, and adherence. Too early for full efficacy but trends emerge. Adjust doses if tolerated but inadequate response.

Week 8: Evaluate full response. If minimal improvement, consider switching rather than prolonging inadequate trial. If partial response, optimize dose or augment.

Months 3, 6, 12: Monitor sustained response, emerging side effects, and adherence. Many patients discontinue during this period without regular contact. Address any functional impairments from medications.

**Side effect screening tools** systematize assessment preventing missed problems:

Sexual function screening (ask all patients on SSRIs/SNRIs):

- "Many people experience sexual changes on these medications. Have you noticed any differences in interest, arousal, or satisfaction?"
- Document baseline function before starting
- Use rating scales for research or unclear cases
- Address proactively rather than waiting for complaints

Weight and metabolic screening:

- Weight at every visit (same scale, same time)
- Waist circumference quarterly with antipsychotics
- Ask about appetite changes, carbohydrate cravings
- Review diet and exercise habits
- Calculate BMI changes

Movement disorder screening:

- Observe gait entering office
- Watch for tremor during conversation
- Ask about restlessness or muscle stiffness
- Perform AIMS exam every 6 months with antipsychotics
- Document any abnormal movements

## Case Example 2: The Missed Monitoring

Jennifer, 28, took quetiapine 400 mg for bipolar disorder for two years without monitoring. She presented requesting weight loss medication after gaining 60 pounds. Review revealed no metabolic labs since initiation.

Immediate testing showed:

- Fasting glucose: 128 mg/dL (prediabetic)

- Triglycerides: 340 mg/dL
- HDL cholesterol: 32 mg/dL
- Waist circumference: 42 inches

This metabolic disaster was preventable with proper monitoring. Interventions:

1. Added metformin 500 mg twice daily
2. Referred to nutritionist
3. Started exercise program
4. Discussed switching to lurasidone
5. Implemented quarterly monitoring

Six months later: 20-pound weight loss, normalized glucose, improving lipids. Jennifer reflected: "I wish someone had warned me and checked labs earlier. I thought weight gain was my fault for lack of willpower."

## Patient Education Templates

Clear, consistent patient education improves adherence and outcomes. These templates provide starting points for common educational needs, adaptable to individual situations.

**Medication information sheets** should include:

What this medication does: Use simple analogies patients understand. "This medication helps your brain's communication system work more smoothly, like oil in an engine." Avoid complex neuroscience that confuses rather than clarifies.

How to take it: Specify timing, food requirements, and what to do if doses are missed. "Take every morning with breakfast. If you forget, take as soon as you remember unless it's almost time for the next dose—never double up."

Timeline for improvement: Set realistic expectations. "Most people notice some changes by 2-3 weeks, but full benefits take 6-8 weeks.

Keep taking it even if you don't feel different right away—it's working behind the scenes."

Common side effects and management: Normalize expected effects. "You might feel queasy the first week—this usually passes. Taking with food helps. Some people feel more anxious initially before feeling better. Contact us if side effects interfere with daily life."

Warning signs requiring immediate attention: Be specific. "Call immediately for: fever with confusion and muscle stiffness, thoughts of self-harm, severe rash especially with mouth sores, or chest pain with irregular heartbeat."

**Side effect diaries** track patterns:

Daily tracking form including:

- Medication taken (time, dose)
- Side effects experienced (rate severity 1-10)
- Timing of side effects
- What helped or made worse
- Impact on daily activities
- Questions for next appointment

Weekly summary to identify patterns:

- Most bothersome side effects
- Times of day worse/better
- Relationship to doses
- Overall trajectory (improving/worsening)

This documentation helps clinicians differentiate temporary adjustment effects from persistent problems requiring intervention.

**Adherence tracking tools** identify problems early:

Simple calendar marking: Check off each dose taken. Visual representation shows patterns—weekend misses, evening doses forgotten, gradual decline in adherence.

Smartphone apps providing:

- Medication reminders
- Adherence statistics
- Mood tracking
- Side effect logs
- Reports for appointments

Pharmacy refill tracking: Calculate days supply versus refill dates. Late refills suggest non-adherence. Some pharmacies provide adherence reports.

## Case Example 3: The Educational Success

Mark, 45, failed multiple antidepressants due to "intolerable side effects." Review revealed he stopped each within days of starting due to expected adjustment effects nobody explained.

Comprehensive education provided:

1. Written timeline of expected effects
2. Side effect diary with severity rating
3. Clear explanation of adjustment period
4. Daily text check-ins first week
5. Emphasis on contacting clinic before stopping

Starting sertraline with this support:

- Day 3: "Nausea severity 6/10, but I know it's temporary"
- Week 1: "Anxiety worse but you warned me—sticking with it"
- Week 3: "Side effects mostly gone, mood maybe better?"
- Week 8: "I can't believe I feel normal again"

Mark succeeded through education and support rather than medication changes. "Nobody ever explained medications properly before. I thought feeling worse meant they weren't working."

# Emergency Contact Protocols

Clear protocols for emergency situations reduce anxiety and improve outcomes. Patients and families need specific guidance about when to worry and what actions to take.

**When to call the prescriber** (next business day):

- New side effects interfering with function
- Partial improvement plateauing
- Medication questions or concerns
- Need for refills or dose adjustments
- Missed doses questions
- Drug interaction concerns

**When to call the prescriber urgently** (same day):

- Suicidal thoughts without immediate plan
- Significant mood changes (mania/severe depression)
- Confusion or memory problems
- Severe side effects (tremor, rash, vision changes)
- Falls or near-falls
- Pregnancy discovery while on medications

**When to go to the ER** immediately:

- Suicidal thoughts with plan or intent
- Suicide attempt or self-harm
- Severe confusion with fever and muscle rigidity
- Chest pain or irregular heartbeat
- Seizures
- Severe allergic reaction (swelling, breathing problems)
- Overdose (intentional or accidental)

**Poison control information**: National helpline 1-800-222-1222 available 24/7 for:

- Accidental overdoses

- Medication identification
- Interaction questions
- Preliminary guidance while awaiting medical care

Additional resources include SAMHSA's National Helpline (1-800-662-4357) for mental health and substance use crisis support, available 24/7 with free, confidential treatment referrals and information services (133).

## Building Your Personal Reference System

These references provide starting points, but effective practice requires personalizing resources to your specific needs and patient population. Create your own quick references including:

- Commonly used medication combinations
- Local pharmacy formulary restrictions
- Preferred specialists for referrals
- Community resources for patients
- Personal prescribing patterns and outcomes

Update references regularly as guidelines change and new evidence emerges. What matters isn't having perfect knowledge but knowing where to find accurate information quickly when needed.

The goal remains helping patients achieve their best possible outcomes through informed, systematic medication management. These tools support but don't replace clinical judgment, therapeutic relationships, and individualized care that defines excellent psychiatric practice.

### Key Takeaways

- Quick reference materials transform complex pharmacology into practical clinical tools
- Medication comparison charts highlight key differences guiding selection decisions

- Starting doses vary significantly based on age, anxiety level, and medical complexity
- Systematic monitoring schedules prevent serious complications while avoiding excessive testing
- Patient education templates improve adherence through clear, consistent information
- Side effect tracking helps differentiate temporary adjustment from persistent problems
- Emergency protocols reduce anxiety by providing specific action guidance
- Personal reference systems should be customized to individual practice patterns
- Regular updates keep references current with evolving evidence
- Tools support but never replace clinical judgment and therapeutic relationships

# Reference

1. Stahl, S. M. (2021). Stahl's essential psychopharmacology: Neuroscientific basis and practical applications (5th ed.). Cambridge University Press.
2. Howes, O. D., & Kapur, S. (2009). The dopamine hypothesis of schizophrenia: Version III—The final common pathway. Schizophrenia Bulletin, 35(3), 549-562.
3. Moret, C., & Briley, M. (2011). The importance of norepinephrine in depression. Neuropsychiatric Disease and Treatment, 7(Suppl 1), 9-13.
4. Sigel, E., & Steinmann, M. E. (2012). Structure, function, and modulation of GABA-A receptors. Journal of Biological Chemistry, 287(48), 40224-40231.
5. Sanacora, G., Treccani, G., & Popoli, M. (2012). Towards a glutamate hypothesis of depression. Neuropharmacology, 62(1), 63-77.
6. Cipriani, A., Furukawa, T. A., Salanti, G., et al. (2018). Comparative efficacy and acceptability of 21 antidepressant drugs for the acute treatment of adults with major depressive disorder. The Lancet, 391(10128), 1357-1366.
7. Seeman, P. (2010). Dopamine D2 receptors as treatment targets in schizophrenia. Clinical Schizophrenia & Related Psychoses, 4(1), 56-73.
8. Shulman, K. I., Herrmann, N., & Walker, S. E. (2013). Current place of monoamine oxidase inhibitors in the treatment of depression. CNS Drugs, 27(10), 789-797.
9. Olfson, M., Marcus, S. C., & Pincus, H. A. (2009). Trends in office-based psychiatric practice. American Journal of Psychiatry, 156(3), 451-457.
10. Riba, M. B., & Balon, R. (2018). Competency in combining pharmacotherapy and psychotherapy: Integrated and split treatment. American Psychiatric Association Publishing.
11. Machado-Vieira, R., Salvadore, G., Luckenbaugh, D. A., et al. (2010). Rapid onset of antidepressant action: A new paradigm in the research and treatment of major depressive disorder. Journal of Clinical Psychiatry, 71(4), 425-430.

12. Serretti, A., & Chiesa, A. (2009). Treatment-emergent sexual dysfunction related to antidepressants: A meta-analysis. Journal of Clinical Psychopharmacology, 29(3), 259-266.
13. Boyer, E. W., & Shannon, M. (2005). The serotonin syndrome. New England Journal of Medicine, 352(11), 1112-1120.
14. Makoul, G., & Clayman, M. L. (2006). An integrative model of shared decision making in medical encounters. Patient Education and Counseling, 60(3), 301-312.
15. O'Brien, C. P. (2011). Addiction and dependence in DSM-V. Addiction, 106(5), 866-867.
16. Julius, R. J., Novitsky, M. A., & Dubin, W. R. (2009). Medication adherence: A review of the literature and implications for clinical practice. Journal of Psychiatric Practice, 15(1), 34-44.
17. Hatfield, D. R., & Ogles, B. M. (2007). Why some clinicians use outcome measures and others do not. Administration and Policy in Mental Health, 34(3), 283-291.
18. U.S. Department of Health and Human Services. (2013). Summary of the HIPAA Privacy Rule. Office for Civil Rights.
19. Spina, E., & de Leon, J. (2015). Clinical applications of CYP genotyping in psychiatry. Journal of Neural Transmission, 122(1), 5-28.
20. Preskorn, S. H. (2019). Drug-drug interactions in psychiatric practice: Part IV. Journal of Psychiatric Practice, 25(5), 391-396.
21. Gillman, P. K. (2007). Tricyclic antidepressant pharmacology and therapeutic drug interactions updated. British Journal of Pharmacology, 151(6), 737-748.
22. Fiedorowicz, J. G., & Swartz, K. L. (2004). The role of monoamine oxidase inhibitors in current psychiatric practice. Journal of Psychiatric Practice, 10(4), 239-248.
23. Johannessen, S. I., & Landmark, C. J. (2010). Antiepileptic drug interactions—Principles and clinical implications. Current Neuropharmacology, 8(3), 254-267.
24. Hansten, P. D. (2003). Drug interaction management. Pharmacy World & Science, 25(3), 94-97.
25. Bridge, J. A., Iyengar, S., Salary, C. B., et al. (2007). Clinical response and risk for reported suicidal ideation and suicide

attempts in pediatric antidepressant treatment. JAMA, 297(15), 1683-1696.

26. Correll, C. U., Manu, P., Olshanskiy, V., et al. (2009). Cardiometabolic risk of second-generation antipsychotic medications during first-time use in children and adolescents. JAMA, 302(16), 1765-1773.

27. Kendell, R. E., Chalmers, J. C., & Platz, C. (1987). Epidemiology of puerperal psychoses. British Journal of Psychiatry, 150, 662-673.

28. Cohen, L. S., Altshuler, L. L., Harlow, B. L., et al. (2006). Relapse of major depression during pregnancy in women who maintain or discontinue antidepressant treatment. JAMA, 295(5), 499-507.

29. Mangoni, A. A., & Jackson, S. H. (2004). Age-related changes in pharmacokinetics and pharmacodynamics. British Journal of Clinical Pharmacology, 57(1), 6-14.

30. American Geriatrics Society. (2019). American Geriatrics Society 2019 updated AGS Beers Criteria for potentially inappropriate medication use in older adults. Journal of the American Geriatrics Society, 67(4), 674-694.

31. Beach, S. R., Kostis, W. J., Celano, C. M., et al. (2014). Meta-analysis of selective serotonin reuptake inhibitor-associated QTc prolongation. Journal of Clinical Psychiatry, 75(5), e441-e449.

32. Zevin, S., & Benowitz, N. L. (1999). Drug interactions with tobacco smoking. Clinical Pharmacokinetics, 36(6), 425-438.

33. Ables, A. Z., & Nagubilli, R. (2010). Prevention, recognition, and management of serotonin syndrome. American Family Physician, 81(9), 1139-1142.

34. Dunkley, E. J., Isbister, G. K., Sibbritt, D., et al. (2003). The Hunter Serotonin Toxicity Criteria: Simple and accurate diagnostic decision rules for serotonin toxicity. QJM, 96(9), 635-642.

35. Frank, C. (2008). Recognition and treatment of serotonin syndrome. Canadian Family Physician, 54(7), 988-992.

36. Strawn, J. R., Keck, P. E., & Caroff, S. N. (2007). Neuroleptic malignant syndrome. American Journal of Psychiatry, 164(6), 870-876.

37. Berman, B. D. (2011). Neuroleptic malignant syndrome: A review for neurohospitalists. The Neurohospitalist, 1(1), 41-47.

38. Oruch, R., Pryme, I. F., Engelsen, B. A., & Lund, A. (2017). Neuroleptic malignant syndrome: An easily overlooked neurologic emergency. Neuropsychiatric Disease and Treatment, 13, 161-175.

39. Oruch, R., Elderbi, M. A., Khattab, H. A., et al. (2014). Lithium: A review of pharmacology, clinical uses, and toxicity. European Journal of Pharmacology, 740, 464-473.

40. Baird-Gunning, J., Lea-Henry, T., Hoegberg, L. C., et al. (2017). Lithium poisoning. Journal of Intensive Care Medicine, 32(4), 249-263.

41. Finley, P. R., Warner, M. D., & Peabody, C. A. (1995). Clinical relevance of drug interactions with lithium. Clinical Pharmacokinetics, 29(3), 172-191.

42. Hieronymus, F., Lisinski, A., Nilsson, S., & Eriksson, E. (2018). Efficacy of selective serotonin reuptake inhibitors in the absence of side effects: A mega-analysis of citalopram and paroxetine in adult depression. Molecular Psychiatry, 23(8), 1731-1736.

43. Fluoxetine Hydrochloride. (2021). In LiverTox: Clinical and research information on drug-induced liver injury. National Institute of Diabetes and Digestive and Kidney Diseases.

44. Cipriani, A., La Ferla, T., Furukawa, T. A., et al. (2010). Sertraline versus other antidepressive agents for depression. Cochrane Database of Systematic Reviews, (4), CD006117.

45. Nevels, R. M., Gontkovsky, S. T., & Williams, B. E. (2016). Paroxetine—The antidepressant from hell? Probably not, but caution required. Psychopharmacology Bulletin, 46(1), 77-104.

46. Castro, V. M., Clements, C. C., Murphy, S. N., et al. (2013). QT interval and antidepressant use: A cross-sectional study of electronic health records. BMJ, 346, f288.

47. Figgitt, D. P., & McClellan, K. J. (2000). Fluvoxamine: An updated review of its use in the management of adults with anxiety disorders. Drugs, 60(4), 925-954.

48. Rothmore, J. (2020). Antidepressant-induced sexual dysfunction. Medical Journal of Australia, 212(7), 329-334.

49. Taylor, M. J., Rudkin, L., Bullemor-Day, P., et al. (2013).
Strategies for managing sexual dysfunction induced by
antidepressant medication. Cochrane Database of Systematic
Reviews, (5), CD003382.
50. Davies, J., & Read, J. (2019). A systematic review into the
incidence, severity and duration of antidepressant withdrawal
effects. Addictive Behaviors, 97, 111-121.
51. Gillman, P. K. (2007). Tricyclic antidepressant pharmacology
and therapeutic drug interactions updated. British Journal of
Pharmacology, 151(6), 737-748.
52. Goldstein, D. J., Lu, Y., Detke, M. J., et al. (2005). Duloxetine
vs. placebo in patients with painful diabetic neuropathy. Pain,
116(1-2), 109-118.
53. Muth, E. A., Haskins, J. T., Moyer, J. A., et al. (1986).
Antidepressant biochemical profile of the novel bicyclic
compound Wy-45,030, an ethyl cyclohexanol derivative.
Biochemical Pharmacology, 35(24), 4493-4497.
54. Knadler, M. P., Lobo, E., Chappell, J., & Bergstrom, R.
(2011). Duloxetine: Clinical pharmacokinetics and drug
interactions. Clinical Pharmacokinetics, 50(5), 281-294.
55. Liebowitz, M. R., Tourian, K. A., Hwang, E., & Mele, L.
(2013). A double-blind, randomized, placebo-controlled study
assessing the efficacy and tolerability of desvenlafaxine 10
and 50 mg/day in adult outpatients with major depressive
disorder. BMC Psychiatry, 13, 94.
56. Thase, M. E. (2006). Effects of venlafaxine on blood pressure:
A meta-analysis of original data from 3744 depressed patients.
Journal of Clinical Psychiatry, 67(4), 519-528.
57. Fava, M., Mulroy, R., Alpert, J., et al. (1997). Emergence of
adverse events following discontinuation of treatment with
extended-release venlafaxine. American Journal of Psychiatry,
154(12), 1760-1762.
58. Bupropion. (2016). In Wikipedia. Retrieved from
https://en.wikipedia.org/wiki/Bupropion.
59. Clayton, A. H., Croft, H. A., & Handiwala, L. (2014).
Antidepressants and sexual dysfunction: Mechanisms and
clinical implications. Postgraduate Medicine, 126(2), 91-99.
60. Gadde, K. M., Parker, C. B., Maner, L. G., et al. (2001).
Bupropion for weight loss: An investigation of efficacy and

tolerability in overweight and obese women. Obesity Research, 9(9), 544-551.

61. Dunner, D. L., Zisook, S., Billow, A. A., et al. (1998). A prospective safety surveillance study for bupropion sustained-release in the treatment of depression. Journal of Clinical Psychiatry, 59(7), 366-373.

62. Anttila, S. A., & Leinonen, E. V. (2001). A review of the pharmacological and clinical profile of mirtazapine. CNS Drug Reviews, 7(3), 249-264.

63. Fawcett, J., & Barkin, R. L. (1998). A meta-analysis of eight randomized, double-blind, controlled clinical trials of mirtazapine for the treatment of patients with major depression and symptoms of anxiety. Journal of Clinical Psychiatry, 59(3), 123-127.

64. Blier, P., Ward, H. E., Tremblay, P., et al. (2010). Combination of antidepressant medications from treatment initiation for major depressive disorder. American Journal of Psychiatry, 167(3), 281-288.

65. Gillman, P. K. (2007). Tricyclic antidepressant pharmacology and therapeutic drug interactions updated. British Journal of Pharmacology, 151(6), 737-748.

66. Anderson, I. M. (2000). Selective serotonin reuptake inhibitors versus tricyclic antidepressants: A meta-analysis of efficacy and tolerability. Journal of Affective Disorders, 58(1), 19-36.

67. Hiemke, C., Bergemann, N., Clement, H. W., et al. (2018). Consensus guidelines for therapeutic drug monitoring in neuropsychopharmacology. Pharmacopsychiatry, 51(1-2), 9-62.

68. Tricyclic Antidepressants. (2022). Cleveland Clinic. Retrieved from https://my.clevelandclinic.org/health/treatments/25146-tricyclic-antidepressants.

69. Shulman, K. I., Herrmann, N., & Walker, S. E. (2013). Current place of monoamine oxidase inhibitors in the treatment of depression. CNS Drugs, 27(10), 789-797.

70. Clinically Relevant Drug Interactions with Monoamine Oxidase Inhibitors. (2022). PubMed Central. Retrieved from https://pmc.ncbi.nlm.nih.gov/articles/PMC9680847/.

71. Monoamine Oxidase Inhibitors (MAOI). (2023). NCBI StatPearls. Retrieved from https://www.ncbi.nlm.nih.gov/books/NBK539848/.

72. Malhi, G. S., Tanious, M., Das, P., et al. (2013). Potential mechanisms of action of lithium in bipolar disorder. CNS Drugs, 27(2), 135-153.

73. Alda, M. (2015). Lithium in the treatment of bipolar disorder: Pharmacology and pharmacogenetics. Molecular Psychiatry, 20(6), 661-670.

74. Grandjean, E. M., & Aubry, J. M. (2009). Lithium: Updated human knowledge using an evidence-based approach. CNS Drugs, 23(5), 397-418.

75. Example Lithium Monitoring Plan. (2023). University of Florida. Retrieved from https://dcf.psychiatry.ufl.edu/submission-support/commonly-submitted-medication-information/example-lithium-monitoring-plan/.

76. Ott, M., Stegmayr, B., Salander Renberg, E., & Werneke, U. (2016). Lithium intoxication: Incidence, clinical course and renal function. Journal of Psychopharmacology, 30(10), 1008-1019.

77. Finley, P. R., Warner, M. D., & Peabody, C. A. (1995). Clinical relevance of drug interactions with lithium. Clinical Pharmacokinetics, 29(3), 172-191.

78. Bowden, C. L., & Singh, V. (2012). Valproate in bipolar disorder: 2000 onwards. Acta Psychiatrica Scandinavica, 126(Suppl 446), 13-20.

79. Target Valproic Acid Levels for Bipolar Disorder. (2023). Healthline. Retrieved from https://www.healthline.com/health/bipolar-disorder/valproic-acid-levels-for-bipolar.

80. Valproic Acid and Sodium Valproate Monitoring. (2023). Specialist Pharmacy Service. Retrieved from https://www.sps.nhs.uk/monitorings/valproic-acid-and-sodium-valproate-monitoring/.

81. Geddes, J. R., Calabrese, J. R., & Goodwin, G. M. (2009). Lamotrigine for treatment of bipolar depression. British Journal of Psychiatry, 194(1), 4-9.

82. Ketter, T. A., Greist, J. H., Graham, J. A., et al. (2006). The effect of dermatologic precautions on the incidence of rash with addition of lamotrigine in the treatment of bipolar I disorder. Journal of Clinical Psychiatry, 67(3), 400-406.

83. Mockenhaupt, M., Messenheimer, J., Tennis, P., & Schlingmann, J. (2005). Risk of Stevens-Johnson syndrome and toxic epidermal necrolysis in new users of antiepileptics. Neurology, 64(7), 1134-1138.

84. Brodie, M. J., & Dichter, M. A. (1996). Antiepileptic drugs. New England Journal of Medicine, 334(3), 168-175.

85. Post, R. M., Ketter, T. A., Uhde, T., & Ballenger, J. C. (2007). Thirty years of clinical experience with carbamazepine in the treatment of bipolar illness. CNS Drugs, 21(1), 47-71.

86. Goodwin, G. M., Bowden, C. L., Calabrese, J. R., et al. (2004). A pooled analysis of 2 placebo-controlled 18-month trials of lamotrigine and lithium maintenance in bipolar I disorder. Journal of Clinical Psychiatry, 65(3), 432-441.

87. Lindström, L., Lindström, E., Nilsson, M., & Höistad, M. (2017). Maintenance therapy with second generation antipsychotics for bipolar disorder. Acta Psychiatrica Scandinavica, 136(3), 269-280.

88. Kapur, S., & Mamo, D. (2003). Half a century of antipsychotics and still a central role for dopamine D2 receptors. Progress in Neuro-Psychopharmacology and Biological Psychiatry, 27(7), 1081-1090.

89. Leucht, S., Corves, C., Arbter, D., et al. (2009). Second-generation versus first-generation antipsychotic drugs for schizophrenia. The Lancet, 373(9657), 31-41.

90. Stahl, S. M. (2018). Beyond the dopamine hypothesis of schizophrenia to three neural networks of psychosis. CNS Spectrums, 23(3), 187-191.

91. Seeman, P. (2014). Clozapine, a fast-off-D2 antipsychotic. ACS Chemical Neuroscience, 5(1), 24-29.

92. Mailman, R. B., & Murthy, V. (2010). Third generation antipsychotic drugs: Partial agonism or receptor functional selectivity? Current Pharmaceutical Design, 16(5), 488-501.

93. Yatham, L. N., Kennedy, S. H., Parikh, S. V., et al. (2018). Canadian Network for Mood and Anxiety Treatments (CANMAT) and International Society for Bipolar Disorders

(ISBD) 2018 guidelines for the management of patients with bipolar disorder. Bipolar Disorders, 20(2), 97-170.
94. Zhou, X., Keitner, G. I., Qin, B., et al. (2015). Atypical antipsychotic augmentation for treatment-resistant depression. Journal of Clinical Psychiatry, 76(3), e375-e382.
95. Dold, M., Aigner, M., Lanzenberger, R., & Kasper, S. (2013). Antipsychotic augmentation of serotonin reuptake inhibitors in treatment-resistant obsessive-compulsive disorder. International Journal of Neuropsychopharmacology, 16(3), 557-574.
96. Metabolic Monitoring of Antipsychotic Medications. (2021). NCBI. Retrieved from https://www.ncbi.nlm.nih.gov/pmc/articles/PMC3979051/.
97. Clinical Pearls for Antipsychotic Induced Metabolic Syndrome. (2021). PubMed Central. Retrieved from https://pmc.ncbi.nlm.nih.gov/articles/PMC8582768/.
98. de Silva, V. A., Suraweera, C., Ratnatunga, S. S., et al. (2016). Metformin in prevention and treatment of antipsychotic induced weight gain. BMC Psychiatry, 16, 341.
99. Dayalu, P., & Chou, K. L. (2008). Antipsychotic-induced extrapyramidal symptoms and their management. Expert Opinion on Pharmacotherapy, 9(9), 1451-1462.
100. Carbon, M., Hsieh, C. H., Kane, J. M., & Correll, C. U. (2017). Tardive dyskinesia prevalence in the period of second-generation antipsychotic use. Journal of Clinical Psychiatry, 78(3), e264-e278.
101. Abnormal Involuntary Movement Scale (AIMS). (2023). Medscape Reference. Retrieved from https://reference.medscape.com/calculator/601/abnormal-involuntary-movement-scale-aims.
102. Sigel, E., & Steinmann, M. E. (2012). Structure, function, and modulation of GABA-A receptors. Journal of Biological Chemistry, 287(48), 40224-40231.
103. Ashton, H. (2005). The diagnosis and management of benzodiazepine dependence. Current Opinion in Psychiatry, 18(3), 249-255.
104. Prescribing and Deprescribing Guidance for Benzodiazepines. (2024). The Lancet. Retrieved from

https://www.thelancet.com/journals/eclinm/article/PIIS2589-5370(24)00086-5/fulltext.

105.     Prescribing Benzodiazepines in General Practice. (2019). PubMed Central. Retrieved from https://pmc.ncbi.nlm.nih.gov/articles/PMC6400612/.

106.     Tapering Patients Off of Benzodiazepines. (2017). American Academy of Family Physicians. Retrieved from https://www.aafp.org/pubs/afp/issues/2017/1101/p606.html.

107.     Wilson, T. K., & Tripp, J. (2023). Buspirone. In StatPearls. StatPearls Publishing.

108.     Hydroxyzine Alternatives for Anxiety. (2023). Talkspace. Retrieved from https://www.talkspace.com/blog/hydroxyzine-alternatives/.

109.     Steenen, S. A., van Wijk, A. J., van der Heijden, G. J., et al. (2016). Propranolol for the treatment of anxiety disorders. Journal of Psychopharmacology, 30(2), 128-139.

110.     Evoy, K. E., Morrison, M. D., & Saklad, S. R. (2017). Abuse and misuse of pregabalin and gabapentin. Drugs, 77(4), 403-426.

111.     Faraone, S. V. (2018). The pharmacology of amphetamine and methylphenidate. Neuroscience & Biobehavioral Reviews, 87, 255-270.

112.     The Pharmacology of Amphetamine and Methylphenidate. (2021). PubMed Central. Retrieved from https://pmc.ncbi.nlm.nih.gov/articles/PMC8063758/.

113.     Methylphenidate ADHD Medication. (2023). ADDitude Magazine. Retrieved from https://www.additudemag.com/medication/methylphenidate/.

114.     ADHD Risk Reduction. (2023). AAFP. Retrieved from https://www.aafp.org/family-physician/patient-care/prevention-wellness/emotional-wellbeing/adhd-toolkit/risk-reduction.html.

115.     Non-stimulants for Adult ADHD. (2023). University of Washington. Retrieved from https://pcl.psychiatry.uw.edu/non-stimulants-for-adult-adhd/.

116.     Cortese, S., Adamo, N., Del Giovane, C., et al. (2018). Comparative efficacy and tolerability of medications for attention-deficit hyperactivity disorder in children, adolescents, and adults. The Lancet Psychiatry, 5(9), 727-738.

117.     Z-Drug Overview. (2023). ScienceDirect. Retrieved from https://www.sciencedirect.com/topics/neuroscience/z-drug.

118.     Taking Z-drugs for Insomnia: Know the Risks. (2023). FDA. Retrieved from https://www.fda.gov/consumers/consumer-updates/taking-z-drugs-insomnia-know-risks.

119.     Alzheimer Dementia: Starting, Stopping Drug Therapy. (2023). Cleveland Clinic. Retrieved from https://consultqd.clevelandclinic.org/alzheimer-dementia-starting-stopping-drug-therapy.

120.     Alzheimer Dementia Treatment Guidelines. (2018). Cleveland Clinic Journal of Medicine. Retrieved from https://www.ccjm.org/content/85/3/209.

121.     Spina, E., & de Leon, J. (2015). Clinical applications of CYP genotyping in psychiatry. Journal of Neural Transmission, 122(1), 5-28.

122.     The Effect of Cytochrome P450 Metabolism on Drug Response, Interactions, and Adverse Effects. (2007). American Academy of Family Physicians. Retrieved from https://www.aafp.org/pubs/afp/issues/2007/0801/p391.html.

123.     Recognition and Treatment of Serotonin Syndrome. (2008). PubMed Central. Retrieved from https://pmc.ncbi.nlm.nih.gov/articles/PMC2464814/.

124.     Serotonin Syndrome: Preventing, Recognizing, and Treating It. (2016). Cleveland Clinic Journal of Medicine. Retrieved from https://www.ccjm.org/content/83/11/810.

125.     QT Prolonging Drugs. (2023). NCBI StatPearls. Retrieved from https://www.ncbi.nlm.nih.gov/books/NBK534864/.

126.     Cohen, L. S., Altshuler, L. L., Harlow, B. L., et al. (2006). Relapse of major depression during pregnancy in women who maintain or discontinue antidepressant treatment. JAMA, 295(5), 499-507.

127.     Bridge, J. A., Iyengar, S., Salary, C. B., et al. (2007). Clinical response and risk for reported suicidal ideation and suicide attempts in pediatric antidepressant treatment. JAMA, 297(15), 1683-1696.

128.     American Geriatrics Society. (2019). American Geriatrics Society 2019 updated AGS Beers Criteria for potentially inappropriate medication use in older adults. Journal of the American Geriatrics Society, 67(4), 674-694.

129.     Should Melatonin Be Used as a Sleeping Aid for Elderly People? (2019). PubMed Central. Retrieved from https://pmc.ncbi.nlm.nih.gov/articles/PMC6699865/.

130.     Treatment-Resistant Depression. (2023). Mayo Clinic. Retrieved from https://www.mayoclinic.org/diseases-conditions/depression/in-depth/treatment-resistant-depression/art-20044324.

131.     Improving Medication Adherence for Chronic Disease Management. (2017). CDC. Retrieved from https://www.cdc.gov/mmwr/volumes/66/wr/mm6645a2.htm.

132.     Cultural Assessment and Treatment of Psychiatric Patients. (2023). NCBI. Retrieved from https://www.ncbi.nlm.nih.gov/books/NBK482311/.

133.     National Helpline for Mental Health, Drug, Alcohol Issues. (2023). SAMHSA. Retrieved from https://www.samhsa.gov/find-help/helplines/national-helpline.

www.ingramcontent.com/pod-product-compliance
Lightning Source LLC
Chambersburg PA
CBHW070805290326
41931CB00011BA/2138